Breast Reconstruction – Your Choice

BREAST RECONSTRUCTION

YOUR
CHOICE

Dick Rainsbury

Consultant Surgeon and Director of Breast Unit
Royal Hampshire County Hospital

Virginia Straker

Researcher, Winchester & Eastleigh NHS Healthcare Trust
and former Senior Breast Care Specialist Nurse
Royal Hampshire County Hospital

CLASS PUBLISHING · LONDON

Text © Dick Rainsbury and Virginia Straker, 2008
Typography © Class Publishing (London) Ltd 2008

Printing history
First published 2008

The information presented in this book is accurate and current to the best of the authors' knowledge. The authors and publisher, however, make no guarantee as to, and assume no responsibility for, the correctness, sufficiency or completeness of such information or recommendation. The reader is advised to consult a doctor regarding all aspects of individual health care.

The author and publishers welcome feedback from the users of this book. Please contact the publishers.

Class Publishing, Barb House, Barb Mews, London W6 7PA, UK
Telephone: 020 7371 2119
Fax: 020 7371 2878
email: post@class.co.uk
Visit our website – www.class.co.uk

A CIP catalogue record for this book is available from the British Library

ISBN: 978 1 85959 197 0

Edited by Caroline Taylor

Designed and typeset by Ray Rich

Illustrations by David Woodroffe

Index by Vicki Robinson

Printed and bound in Slovenia by Korotan

Contents

Acknowledgements vii

Preface viii

Foreword ix

Contributors x

1   **Breast reconstruction – your choice** 1
Dick Rainsbury

2   **What is breast reconstruction?** 5
Dick Rainsbury

3   **Subpectoral reconstruction and implants** 23
Chris Khoo

4   **Reconstruction with a latissimus dorsi (LD) flap** ... 44
     Implant-based LD reconstruction 45
     Dick Rainsbury
     Autologous LD flap reconstruction 61
     Eva Weiler-Mithoff

5   **Reconstruction with a transverse rectus abdominus
myocutaneous (TRAM) flap** 73
     Pedicled TRAM flap reconstruction 73
     Andrew Baildam
     Free TRAM flap reconstruction (DIEP flap) 85
     Eva Weiler-Mithoff

6   **Reconstruction after partial mastectomy** 102
Dick Rainsbury

7   **Reconstruction of the nipple and areola** 115
Venkat V. Ramakrishnan and Diana E.M. Slade-Sharman

8   **Surgery on your other breast** 128
Andrew D. Baildam

9   **Possible complications after breast reconstruction** ... 137
Siobhan Laws

10 Will my reconstruction be affected by my breast cancer treatment? 146
Virginia Hall

11 'Risk-reducing' mastectomy and reconstruction for high genetic risk 151
Diana M. Eccles

12 Getting ready for breast reconstruction 161
Lyn Booth

13 Physiotherapy and rehabilitation after breast reconstruction 169
Catriona Futter

14 Anxieties and concerns about breast reconstruction 180
Diana Harcourt

15 Mastectomy without reconstruction 191
Virginia Straker

16 Getting all your information together quickly 203
Virginia Straker

17 Final comments – Would I do it again? 209
Virginia Straker

Useful contacts and sources of information 215

Glossary 221

Index 227

Acknowledgements

The editors would like to thank the following for their invaluable help with the production of this book: Mentor Medical Systems Limited and The Winchester Cancer Research Trust for their generous sponsorship; the patients who gave their time and spoke honestly and thoughtfully about their experiences in the hope that their stories would help others in the future; Helen Gooch for her patient and cheerful secretarial and administrative support; David Woodroffe for his illustrations; Paul Braham for his help with the photographs; Amoena (UK) Ltd for the use of a photograph; and Francis Pott for supporting and encouraging the project.

Preface

In 1999 I faced my biggest challenge – breast cancer and a bilateral mastectomy. I thought my world had ended: it was unfair, I was angry and I needed information. I thought that understanding a little bit about the disease would help me beat it. I was lucky enough to meet a brilliant surgeon, a man who helped me do just that. I devoured book after book, trawled the internet and spoke to incredible women who had faced cancer – my bosom buddies, as they were known. At a time when you feel vulnerable there are very difficult decisions to be made. For me one of them was whether to have breast reconstruction or not. It didn't take me long to decide that I wanted to, but what did it involve? Dick Rainsbury patiently explained the various procedures that would be suitable for me. It was some months after my successful op that I suggested he write a book to explain to women and their partners what breast reconstruction is all about – a book that would have all the information you need, at your fingertips. This he has done, with the aid of Virginia Straker. Just as I was helped, I hope this book will help many others. Thank you both for doing this.

Sally Taylor
TV Presenter

Foreword

It's 20 December 2006. I already know I have breast cancer, but have just gone through a barrage of tests to determine the size of the invader and what type of surgery will be necessary. My right breast feels battered and bruised, a description that would equally fit my state of mind.

'I'm afraid it will have to be a mastectomy.' My surgical oncologist sounds warm and regretful. He must have delivered this news thousands of times to so many women, but he manages to sound as if his concern is only for me. He's good at his job. But all I want to do is fix a date for the op and get out of there, absorb the awful news, grieve and then get on with the inevitable. There is more though. 'We need to discuss reconstruction', he says. For a moment I think he's mad and tell him to just get rid of the cancer by whatever means necessary. 'No,' he persists, 'I can't promise to make you look perfect naked.' For the first time in several days I feel a sense of humour returning. 'I haven't looked perfect naked for quite some time, don't worry about it.' 'No,' he says, 'take me seriously. I can help you feel confident in your clothes and we need to make a decision now because it will affect the way I carry out the operation.' He carefully explains about retaining skin, inserting tissue expanders, different forms of reconstruction that we can decide about later, but a yes or no to tissue expansion is what he needs to know before I give myself up to his scalpel. I agree.

In the end I decided against any reconstruction involving surgery on other parts of my body – back or stomach – I felt I'd been through enough. I agreed to the insertion of an implant and together we ruled out reduction of the other side. I worked on the principle 'If it ain't broke, why fix it?' and had some concerns that surgery on a healthy breast may cause lack of feeling in the remaining nipple. I'd rather enjoyed the sensation in the past and saw no good reason to lose the potential for further pleasure.

So, I remain lopsided and fill my bra with a prosthesis, which is light and unobtrusive, and the reconstructed breast at least gives me some cleavage in a lowish neck. Most importantly, I was given the facts and time to make the choice that was right for me. What more could we ask?

Jenni Murray
Writer and Broadcaster

Contributors

Mr Andrew D. Baildam MD FRCS
Consultant Oncoplastic and Breast Surgeon and Honorary Senior
Lecturer in Surgical Oncology, The Nightingale Centre,
University Hospital of South Manchester, Southmoor Road,
Wythenshawe, Manchester M23 9LT

Ms Lyn Booth SRN BSc (Hons) Nursing
Breast Care Specialist Nurse, Royal Hampshire County Hospital,
Romsey Road, Winchester, Hampshire SO22 5DG

Professor Diana M. Eccles MD FRCP
Professor of Cancer Genetics and Honorary Consultant in
Clinical Genetics, Wessex Clinical Genetics Service,
Level G Princess Anne Hospital, Southampton SO16 6YA

Mrs Catriona Futter BSc MPhil MCSP
Senior Physiotherapist, Physiotherapy Department,
Canniesburn Plastic Surgery Unit, Jubilee Building,
Glasgow Royal Infirmary, 84 Castle Street, Glasgow G4 0SF

Dr Virginia Hall FRCR
Consultant in Clinical Oncology, Southampton General Hospital,
Tremona Road, Southampton SO16 6YD

Dr Diana Harcourt PhD MSc BSc (Hons)
Reader in Health Psychology and Co-Director of the Centre for
Appearance Research, University of the West of England,
Coldharbour Lane, Frenchay, Bristol BS16 1QY

Mr Chris Khoo FRCS
Consultant Plastic Surgeon, Bakers Barn, Touchen End,
Maidenhead, Berkshire SL6 3LD

Ms Siobhan Laws MBBS FRCS DM
Consultant Breast and General Surgeon, Surgical Unit Office,
MP82, Royal Hampshire County Hospital, Romsey Road,
Winchester, Hampshire SO22 5DG

Mr Dick Rainsbury BSc MS FRCS

Consultant Oncoplastic Breast Surgeon and Director of
Education, Royal College of Surgeons of England,
The Breast Unit, Royal Hampshire County Hospital,
Romsey Road, Winchester, Hampshire SO22 5DG

Mr Venkat V. Ramakrishnan MS FRCS FRACS

Consultant Plastic Surgeon, St Andrew's Centre for Plastic and
Reconstructive Surgery, Court Road, Broomfield, Chelmsford,
Essex CM1 7ET

**Ms Diana E.M. Slade-Sharman FRCS Plast MSc FRCS Eng
BSc MBBS**

Specialist Registrar in Plastic Surgery, Matching House,
7 Pye Gardens, Bishop's Stortford, Hertfordshire CM23 2GU

Ms Virginia Straker SRN

c/o Winchester and Andover Breast Unit, Royal Hampshire
County Hospital, Romsey Road, Winchester, Hampshire
SO22 5DG

Mrs Eva Weiler-Mithoff FRCS Ed FRCS Glas, Plast

Consultant Plastic Surgeon, Canniesburn Plastic Surgery Unit,
Jubilee Building, Glasgow Royal Infirmary, 84 Castle Street,
Glasgow G4 0SF

1

Breast reconstruction – your choice

- It's now possible to rebuild a breast which looks just like the one that's been removed.

- Having reconstruction at the same time as your mastectomy is often the best option.

- With some types of breast cancer, it's better to delay reconstruction until all the treatment is finished.

- This book is based around the experiences of more than sixty women who made a choice about breast reconstruction.

'I am afraid to tell you you have got breast cancer and you're going to need a mastectomy.'

Hundreds of women hear these words every week in the UK, launching them headlong into a scary and unfamiliar world, filled with doubts, uncertainties and fear of the unknown. Scores of questions rush to mind. How bad is the cancer? Will I live? Will it be painful? Will I need chemotherapy? What about my family and my children? Have I passed it on? How long will I have to wait? Why me?

And then as the word 'mastectomy' sinks in, other thoughts raise their ugly heads. Is it that bad? Must I really lose my breast? How will it feel? Will people know? Will I ever look the same again?

This book is based around the very personal experiences of more than sixty women, from five major centres in the UK, who have faced mastectomy and have chosen to have a breast reconstruction – an operation to rebuild the breast and restore what disease and surgery have taken away. Their own words are used to track a journey starting

1

from the moment of diagnosis through to surgery and finally on to full recovery. It is hoped that by following their journey the reader will be helped to understand the steps along the way and to ask the most important questions at each stage of their treatment.

What is breast reconstruction?

What does breast reconstruction mean? How can an organ as complicated as the breast be 'recreated' and when can this be done? These are very important questions that often go unasked and unanswered because those looking after you may think you know the answers already – but very often you don't. Put simply, breast reconstruction is an operation in which the breast that has been taken away is replaced with something that looks like the real thing. With modern techniques surgeons can make a new breast that looks extremely lifelike – so much so that you may have to look very hard indeed to spot the difference. This is because some patients have their whole breast removed through such a small cut around the nipple that the surgeon can rebuild the new breast inside the natural skin pocket. This can leave just a tiny and almost invisible scar around the edge of the nipple.

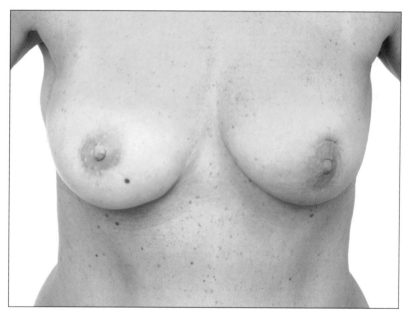

Right mastectomy and reconstruction with tummy tissue leaving invisible scars

But not every patient is suitable for this approach. The final appearance of the new breast will depend on many factors, including the type of mastectomy, the length of the scars, the type of reconstruction, the skill of the surgeon and whether your reconstruction is done at the same time as your mastectomy. And even though the breast may look normal, it won't *feel* like a normal breast, it won't *work* like a normal breast and it won't even move like a normal breast. Depending on what kind of reconstruction you chose, the new breast will usually feel numb in the middle. This feeling is most intense in the early days after surgery, but gradually some of the sensation returns as the nerves grow back, starting around the edges of your new breast. Your new breast may also feel colder than the other side, particularly after a swim in cold water.

Often the nipple will be removed and although it can be reconstructed, it won't have any sensation and won't respond to stimulation. And because all the glandular tissue has been removed, it won't change with the menstrual cycle, it can't make milk, and it may not change shape in the same way as your remaining breast as you get older. But your new breast will look normal to those around you. If the very latest techniques are used you'll be able to feel confident wearing a low neckline, a swimsuit or even when topless. For many women, this is a big improvement to the alternative – a mastectomy scar and an external prosthesis. For others, the extra surgery, longer recovery and the higher risk of complications are too great a price to pay. They may decide that reconstruction is not for them.

One of the most important unasked questions about breast reconstruction is, 'When can it be done?' All too often you don't think about asking or don't know about the possibility, and there are so many other important things going through your mind before you have to come in for surgery. It's one question too many. But if you would like to consider reconstruction, then the time to ask your surgeon and your team is before you have your mastectomy. This is because it may be possible to rebuild your breast at the same time as your cancer surgery is carried out. This will depend on so many things – your choice, your health, your tumour, your surgeon and the type of treatment planned after your operation. But if you don't ask the question, you may simply miss a big opportunity to have this type of surgery. And by having your breast reconstructed during your mastectomy operation (immediate breast reconstruction), you'll cut down on the number of operations, the length of your convalescence and time off work. And you'll also avoid much of the distress experienced by women who lose a breast as a result of a mastectomy.

But not every patient is suitable for immediate breast reconstruction, and even those who are often find it difficult to make a decision in the few days between hearing the diagnosis and their admission to hospital for surgery. Other patients may be referred to units that are not able to perform immediate breast reconstruction – as a result, they may choose to put off a decision until their treatment has been completed.

This book has been written with one aim in mind – to explain your options and to provide accurate, up-to-date information and advice to steer you through the increasingly bewildering world of breast reconstruction. The time, effort and personal accounts provided freely by so many women in the following pages are a testimony to the increasing importance of breast reconstruction to women in the UK today. The editors would like to thank all of these women, and also those who have given permission to have their photographs included throughout the book.

2 What is breast reconstruction?

- **Choosing breast reconstruction is a very important decision to make.**
- **It can be done straight away or later on.**
- **Get all the advice you can before making up your mind.**
- **Don't go ahead if you're not certain.**
- **A reconstructed breast matures over several months.**
- **Reconstruction often requires more than one operation.**

People talk about breast reconstruction, but how on earth can you rebuild such a complicated part of your body? There are now some very modern techniques used by surgeons to rebuild a breast that is soft and that moves and looks like the real thing. But it can't produce milk and it is usually quite numb, especially around the nipple and the middle part of the breast. So it may look almost exactly like your other breast, but it is only a replica – it's not the real thing. But many women who have a reconstruction get on with life without any restrictions on what they wear, playing sport or personal relationships. This is because their new breast becomes part and parcel of their own body, just like the breast that was taken away.

Choosing whether you're going to have a breast reconstruction is one of the bigger decisions in your life. You've already just been told you need a mastectomy, and maybe a range of other treatments such as chemotherapy, hormone therapy and radiotherapy. And almost in the same sentence, the surgeon talks about breast reconstruction and rattles off a variety of options, using words you've never heard of before. You're anxious and confused. Too much information, too many decisions, too little time. You forget to ask the important questions and before you have time to think, you are sent off to see the breast care nurse. She gives you all the information all over again, and lots of leaflets and booklets to take away.

Eventually you're free to leave, glad to be out of the hospital, and hurry home. But then you realise you have forgotten almost everything they said to you. Questions race through your head. When can it be done? What will it be like? Am I the right person for reconstruction? Will it affect my cancer? Is this a once and for all operation? What are my options? What about the other breast? Is my surgeon experienced?

Let's stand back and take a good long look at these very important questions and concerns to try to help you to understand more about breast reconstruction. Then you'll be in a better position to make a decision that is right for you and those close to you.

When can it be done?

There are two main choices when deciding about the timing of your breast reconstruction. You can have it done at the same time as your mastectomy or partial mastectomy – this is called 'immediate' breast reconstruction. Or you can have your breast rebuilt months or years after your mastectomy – 'delayed' breast reconstruction. If your surgeon recommends that only part of your breast is removed and that the gap left behind should be reconstructed, you may be told that it is better to wait for the pathologist to check your tumour before the gap is rebuilt a few days later. This is a type of immediate breast reconstruction that is now becoming more popular.

So why don't all women who want breast reconstruction decide to have this done at the same time as their mastectomy – surely this is better all round? This is a really key question, opening the way to all the other questions you may want to ask. And like so many important questions, it is not fair to expect you to be able to make a decision until you've had a chance to look at all the arguments. When you have a mastectomy, you have three choices to make about breast reconstruction – should you have it straight away, should it be delayed or should you have it at all? So let's have a good look at the main advantages and disadvantages you need to know about to help you make your mind up.

Choosing immediate breast reconstruction

Advantages

- Your breast is removed and reconstructed all at the same time, so you don't have to go through the distressing experience of losing your breast.

- You avoid having to have two major operations, as they are both carried out by one or two teams of surgeons under the same anaesthetic.

- You have one visit to the hospital, one anaesthetic, one period of recovery and one stretch of time off work.

- Your scars are usually much smaller and can be hidden away more easily.

- The appearance of your breast is usually more natural as nearly all of the skin that covers your breast can be saved. This helps the surgeons to shape your new breast, like 'putting jelly back into a jelly mould'.

- You avoid the anxiety and the inconvenience, discomfort and disability of two operations.

- It's much easier for your surgeons as they can plan and integrate everything at the same time, giving you the very best chance of a good cosmetic result.

- It's much easier for your partner, family and friends. They don't have to worry about you having another operation hanging over your head if you decide later to have a delayed reconstruction.

Disdvantages

- You have lots of other things on your mind and may find it very difficult to make such a big decision in a very short timeframe.

- You're naturally upset about your diagnosis and can't think straight.

- You don't have a chance to see what it's like without a reconstruction, to help you decide if you really want to have this further surgery.

- You'll be having more major surgery, with a longer anaesthetic and the risk of more complications.

- Your period of recovery will also be longer than you need after a straightforward mastectomy.

- There's a chance that if you develop complications, any chemotherapy or radiotherapy treatment that the doctors may recommend will be delayed – but the chances of this happening are very small.

- If your doctor decides you need radiotherapy treatment, this can affect the softness and shape of your new breast. One of the problems is that it isn't always possible for your surgeon to know if you are going to need to have radiotherapy until after you've had your mastectomy and they've had a chance to examine all your tissues.

- Unless you're having a mastectomy for 'pre-cancer' (ductal carcinoma in situ – DCIS), there's always a slight chance you'll be advised to have radiotherapy, which in turn may make your reconstructed breast less natural to look at and to touch. More often than not, your surgeon will have a good idea if radiotherapy is going to be needed, and may advise you that a delayed reconstruction would be a more sensible choice.

There's one really important piece of advice if you are thinking about reconstruction. If you really can't make up your mind about whether to go ahead, don't feel cornered into making a snap decision. Ask for more information from your breast care nurse and speak to your own doctor. There are lots of helpful sources of information (pp. 215–219) – one of the most valuable is to speak to other patients who have had to make the same decisions as you. They will tell you about their own experiences and reactions, their recovery, and lots of other things that doctors and nurses won't have experienced themselves.

If you still feel unable to make up your mind, then it's probably wisest *not* to go ahead with a reconstruction. If you feel pressurised to go ahead and things go wrong, you'll wish you had never had it done. You can always have a new breast at a later date once you have had a chance to get over your treatment and return to normal. The timing of breast reconstruction is a very individual choice and there are many different factors in deciding which choice is best for you and your own particular circumstances. These two patients opted for immediate breast reconstruction:

" I am slim and very conscious of my body and wanted to get the best result if I was going to have a mastectomy and breast reconstruction done. I lead a really young lifestyle, going clubbing and dancing, and my body is important to me. "

" I would urge women to go for immediate breast reconstruction if it is offered, because to go back for a reconstruction after mastectomy would be daunting. If you are able to come out of surgery feeling feminine, able to wear nice swimsuits and go into a public changing room without worrying, this is great. Also, I wanted to be able to cuddle my grandchildren and didn't want to be a different shape for them. "

Another two patients felt that delayed reconstruction was the right thing for them:

" I coped very well with the mastectomy. What I didn't like was having to keep putting the plastic thing on every morning and washing it at night. It emphasised the deformity. I thought that there was no way that I could go through life like that. I wanted to have a breast back. I realised how much I had been pushing those feelings back, in order to cope with the diagnosis. "

" I feel that I made the right decision about delaying reconstruction. Things happened so quickly and I don't think I could have made a decision about reconstruction as well at the time. I knew that the opportunity would still be there for me in the future. It was important for me that I wasn't shutting the door on it. "

Finally, if you need another week or two to make up your mind, don't be afraid to ask for more time. It's not going to make the slightest difference to your chances of recovery, and may just be the time you need to be sure you've made the best decision for you.

What will it be like?

" I was just 50 when I was told I needed a mastectomy, but could have a breast reconstruction as well. As I had no previous experience of it, I just could not possibly imagine what a mastectomy or reconstruction would look like. "

Most people have no idea what a reconstructed breast will look like and how it will feel. In today's 'topless' society, this may seem quite strange. It's partly because up until recently, fewer than one in ten women had had breast reconstruction, so there aren't that many women around who have had this done. It's also because it's only recently that new techniques have been developed to help the surgeon to hide the scars of surgery so they become almost invisible. These new techniques can make women much more confident about their shape and appearance. Different kinds of breast reconstruction produce different results. We will talk about these later in this section.

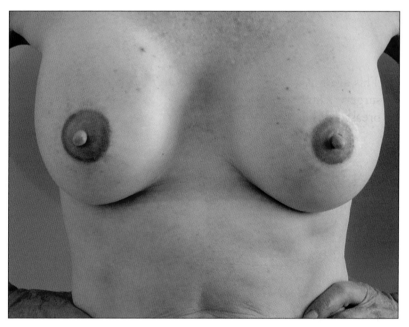

Bilateral mastectomies and immediate reconstruction (nipple reconstruction and tattoo hides the scars)

Let's have a look at some things that you'll probably notice soon after your operation, whatever kind of reconstruction you've had. When you wake up from the anaesthetic and take a look at your reconstructed breast, don't be surprised to find some of these things:

- **Your new breast is a different size to your other breast**

  It may be larger because of swelling and bruising, which will gradually settle down. Some kinds of reconstruction may take up to a year before they reach their final size, so you may need to be patient while these changes are going on. Or your new breast may be smaller if you have chosen to have a reconstruction with a 'tissue expander'. This will be used to enlarge your breast during the early weeks after your operation.

- **It's a different shape compared with your other breast**

  Very often your new breast will look fuller and rounder near the top, but flatter and emptier near the bottom – the reverse of the normal shape of your breast. Don't worry about this. It happens because your surgeon has reconstructed your new breast to look like a younger breast to begin with, knowing that it will gradually move downwards with the effect of gravity. By doing this, it will end up with a much more natural shape in the long run.

- **It feels very firm and unnatural, and doesn't move about like a normal breast**

  This again is completely normal in the early months after your surgery. Once healing and any adjustments are completed, your breast will become softer and will begin to move about like the other side. Major surgery produces a lot of swelling. If an implant or tissue expander was used for your operation, this will increase the swelling further still. You can imagine that if all this swelling is going on in the space that is left behind after removing your breast, your new breast gets blown up a bit like a balloon and can become quite hard. Gradually the swelling drains away and settles down, but you have to be patient while your body adjusts to these changes.

- **The skin of the new breast will feel very numb**

  This is because nearly all of the small nerves to the skin have been cut to remove your breast. You may not notice this until you get home. Some of the feeling will gradually return as the nerves grow back around the edge of your new breast. This can feel very strange while it's going on, and will take twelve to twenty-four months, but the middle area of your new breast will always feel numb. And if you've had an operation which uses a 'flap' for the reconstruction (see pp. 44 and 73), the flap itself, and the skin near where the flap was taken from, will also feel completely numb. So you have to be careful with, for example, hot water bottles, which can burn these areas of skin while you are asleep without you feeling anything at all.

● **Your scars will depend on what kind of reconstruction you've had**
If your reconstruction is done at the same time as your mastectomy, the scars are often in the middle of your new breast and usually very small. If on the other hand you have a delayed reconstruction, the surgeon will often use your mastectomy scar, so the scar will be about the same length as before.

● **If you've had a flap operation, you will notice an 'island' of new skin somewhere in the middle of your breast**
This will be surrounded by a scar, and the island will usually have a slightly different colour and texture from the skin of your breast. This is because it's been removed from another part of your body, such as your back or your tummy. The so-called 'patch' effect will usually become less obvious as time goes by. The scars often become thin white lines over the next year or two. In a small number of people they become red and thickened in the early months. If this happens to you, be patient, as they will nearly always settle down within a couple of years. The same thing may happen to the scars on your back or your tummy if you've had a flap operation.

And finally, it's important to know what you are going to feel like when you come round from your operation.

● Remember you're going to have quite a big operation, depending on the type of reconstruction you've chosen. The surgery may take as little as two hours if it is going to be done using an implant or a tissue expander. A flap operation is more complicated, because tissue has to be moved very carefully from one part of your body to another. This often takes between four and six hours to do and sometimes as long as eight hours.

● When you come round, you'll find you're back on the ward. You may even be on a special ward if you've had a flap operation. This is so that the nurses can check and monitor the blood supply to your flap more closely for the first twelve to twenty-four hours. It shouldn't be painful because the anaesthetist often uses a 'block' to deaden the nerves around the operation. You'll also have a button to press that will deliver medications to help to keep any pain at bay.

- Don't be surprised if you're attached to lots of drips and drains, and a urinary catheter, when you wake up. They are there to replace and measure any fluids lost during or after your surgery, and they'll be removed as soon as your doctors are happy that they aren't needed any more.

- You'll probably be up and about the day after your operation, and your breast team and physiotherapist will help you to get back on your feet as soon as possible. It's likely you will be back home within four or five days.

Am I the right person to have reconstruction?

Almost anyone can have a breast reconstruction, but you need to decide if this is the right thing for you. Your surgeon and your breast team should be able to help you answer part of this question. They will be able to tell you if you're physically fit for the operation and also that it won't be affected badly by any treatment that is planned for you after your surgery. In fact, they won't suggest reconstruction unless they think you are fit enough to have this type of surgery in the first place.

The second part of this question is much more personal, and only you can give an honest answer. You may be the kind of person who can make a quick decision to go ahead as soon as you are offered the choice:

> 66 I was 66 when I was told that I had breast cancer and needed a mastectomy. I was shattered. All my life I had thought that breast cancer was about the worst thing that could happen to me because I would be disfigured. Anything to keep my femininity and be able to present myself to the world as the same person was important. 99

13

But it's important that you don't let your heart lead your head. Although your first reaction is often your final decision, you really need to think about your options and ask lots of questions. Then if things don't turn out the way you wanted, at least you'll know you made a balanced decision.

It's easier in a way if you've already had a mastectomy and are thinking about delayed reconstruction, because you know what it's like and you've got plenty of time to think and to do your own research. And age in itself is no barrier – it's your health and self-motivation that really matters the most:

> " I had worn two prostheses for some time and found them pretty awful. I got the leaflets about reconstruction out again. I thought that reconstruction would be better than working with two prostheses. It didn't even dawn on me that I might not consider reconstruction at 62. "

Will it affect my cancer?

When breast reconstruction was introduced more than 30 years ago, no one knew if it was safe, from the breast cancer point of view. So women had to wait for at least two years after their mastectomy before reconstruction was done. Now things are completely different. Many studies have shown this type of surgery doesn't stimulate the cancer to grow back, it doesn't make it spread, and it doesn't make cancer any more difficult to detect in the few women who develop a recurrence after surgery. So nowadays if you decide to have immediate breast reconstruction it won't affect your cancer in any way. On the other hand, if the treatment of your cancer includes radiotherapy, this can affect the appearance of your reconstruction, so you and your surgeon should discuss this together before you go ahead.

Is this a once and for all operation?

The simple answer to this question for most people is 'no' – for two main reasons:

- It's very difficult to match your remaining breast in one operation. You'll almost certainly need further adjustments to your recon-struction or to your opposite breast if you want a balanced, natural-looking result. These are usually small operations that may be done as a day case and from which you'll have a quick recovery. You may need to have a reduction or an enlargement of your remaining breast, a nipple reconstruction and a tattoo, or an exchange of your implant to get a better shape.

● Later on, as you grow older, your reconstructed breast may not 'age' in appearance as quickly as your own breast. Further adjustments may be needed to bring both breasts into line. And if it's been rebuilt using an implant, this may need to be checked and changed once it's been in place for ten years or more (see p. 45). So like any 'spare part' surgery, further straightforward procedures may be needed to 'service' your reconstruction as time goes by.

What are my options?

There are three very different techniques that your surgeon can use to reconstruct your breast.

● **An implant or tissue expander (an adjustable type of implant)**
This is slipped into the space that lies between your ribs and your pectoralis muscle, which lies behind your breast. This is called a subpectoral reconstruction. It means that your surgeon does not have to create a flap. It also means that most of your breast is made from the implant or expander, and contains little of your own tissue (see p. 29).

● **Combination of an implant or tissue expander together with a muscle flap**
This technique is becoming very popular, and the muscle that is usually chosen comes from your back. The technique is called latissimus dorsi reconstruction. This approach has been used for over 30 years because it's so reliable. After this operation, between a third and a half of your breast is made from your own tissue, and the rest is made from the implant or tissue expander (see p. 45).

● **Building your new breast using all your own tissue without the need for an implant or a tissue expander**
This approach is called autologous reconstruction, which normally uses tissue from the lower part of your tummy – the 'TRAM flap' (see p. 73) or 'DIEP flap' (see p. 85). New techniques are helping surgeons to use other flaps, such as flaps from the buttock or the

inside of the thigh, as well as using a much bigger part of latissimus dorsi (LD) – your back muscle. This is called an autologous latissimus dorsi reconstruction (see p. 61).

When giving you advice about your reconstruction options, your surgeon will make an assessment of you as a person, as well as the treatment you are likely to need. On the one hand, your shape, size, expectations and general health will need to be taken into account. On the other, your surgeon will need to consider your chances of needing radiotherapy after your surgery, which in turn will influence the surgical options. It's important that you ask as many questions as possible at this stage about your different choices – for example, about your hospital stay, your recovery, your scars and the effect of surgery on day-to-day activities and sports. It's also important to find out how the operation will affect you in years to come.

> " I think it would have been helpful if I'd asked a bit more about the long-term effects of reconstruction without an implant, and talked to someone who had had a similar operation. When you are discussing options with the doctor, you need to make it very clear what sort of activities you do and that you wish to be able to carry on with them afterwards. It is important to be able to pick up your life afterwards and carry on. "

So you need to give the doctors and the nurses as much information about yourself as you possibly can. Ask your team if it would be possible to speak to other women who have faced similar choices, and have made different decisions about their surgery.

> " I was offered either latissimus dorsi or a DIEP flap for the breast reconstruction. I made up my mind in two weeks, although I could have had longer. I didn't want to keep putting off the inevitable. It is hard, because you try to cope with the diagnosis of cancer and all the worries that brings, and at the same time try to decide between two different procedures. It is impossible to know what the outcome is going to be. I read as much information as I could get my hands on, and also discussed it with my family. I wondered how on earth I was going to make a decision. I was lucky enough to speak to two women who had the breast reconstruction I was considering. That was very helpful. "

The trouble is that you'll be given an awful lot of information, which you have to try to take on board all at once. So here's a simple list of the important advantages and disadvantages of the three main approaches. It's to help you see how they compare with each other, and to help you ask some key questions.

Subpectoral reconstruction

Advantages

- It's the simplest approach.

- It's the shortest operation.

- It has the quickest recovery.

- There are no scars, except the ones on your breast.

- It has no effects on other parts of your body.

Disadvantages

- There are small risks of infection, haemorrhage and loss of your implant or expander, as well as a poor cosmetic result.

- You'll need several visits to outpatients for tissue expansion to enlarge and shape your breast. These visits will take place over several months.

- It's difficult to achieve a natural shape and position using this technique.

- Only a small amount of your breast is made from your own tissues.

- Your new breast won't mature like a normal breast.

- It won't feel as soft, warm and fleshy as your normal breast.

- As scar tissue forms around the implant or expander, it's easier to feel and may make the breast feel harder than the other side.

- You're more likely to go through further operations to change your implant or expander to adjust your shape, compared with other techniques.

Latissimus dorsi reconstruction using implant or expander

Advantages

- Your new breast will have a natural shape and movement more like your other breast.

- It'll feel soft and warm and fleshy.

- Up to half of your new breast will be made of your own tissue, so it'll feel more normal and will change with your body weight.

- It'll 'mature' like your other breast, and will move down to a lower position as you grow older.

- If scar tissue forms around your implant or expander, it won't be so easy to feel, because it lies quite deeply behind your flap.

- It's unusual to have to do any further operations on your reconstructed breast, but a few women need to have their implant or expander swapped for a new one several years later.

Disadvantages

- It's a major operation, which takes four to six hours to carry out. Your hospital stay and recovery will be longer than after subpectoral reconstruction.

- It's slightly more risky than subpectoral reconstruction because of the flap. This can rarely develop problems with its blood supply, and fluid can collect in the pocket where the flap was taken from on your back.

- You'll have scars on your back as well as on your breast. These are often hidden under your bra strap, but they can show and become thickened.

- You may feel tightness around your chest after your surgery. This can last for a few months.

- You might experience slight weakness when pushing your shoulder back on your reconstructed side. This may have a slight effect on sports such as skiing and rowing because the muscle has been moved to a different position, but it shouldn't affect your normal day-to-day activities.

Autologous reconstruction

Advantages

- Your new breast will have the most natural shape and movement of all reconstructions – because it's all you.

- Like you, it will put on and lose weight, depending on your diet and lifestyle, and will feel soft and warm just like your other breast.

- There's no implant or expander, so once the initial surgery is finished, you shouldn't need any more operations on your reconstruction.

- If you've had a TRAM or DIEP flap, you'll lose quite a lot of your tummy. Some women see this as an added bonus.

Disadvantages

- These are usually the most complex of all reconstruction operations. They can take up to eight hours to do.

- You may have to spend the first few hours of your recovery in a High Dependency Unit. This is to monitor the blood supply to your flap more closely, as it can occasionally get blocked off and require further surgery to clear the blockage.

- Occasionally, the blockage cannot be cleared, which means that the flap dies off and has to be taken away.

- You will have quite a long scar on your tummy, possibly on your back, your leg or your buttock, depending on the type of operation which you've had done (see pp. 63, 75 and 99).

- You may have some weakness in your tummy muscles early on, which will usually improve. There's also a small chance of developing a hernia (bulge) in your tummy later on.

Remember that it's important to ask your surgeon to run through your own choices for reconstruction. Make sure that each of these options has been considered and whether in fact they're all carried out by the team that is treating you. If they're not, then you can ask to be referred on to a team that carries out the operation that appeals to you. Once you've had the operation, it's very difficult to go back and do something different.

❝ I was only given the option of having a Becker tissue expander, but probably could have had a choice of different reconstructions if I had asked more questions. In an ideal world, people should have the chance to consider all the options, as well as seeing people who have had them by the same surgeon. Tissue expansion is a relatively simple process compared with other methods. With hindsight, I did not have enough information to make a balanced judgement. The issues that I did not know about were how much additional surgery I would have, and how long the whole expansion process took. People need to have realistic expectations and understand that the reconstructive process may be a good imitation, but not exactly the same. What is good for one person may not be good for another. ❞

What about the other breast?

There are two important questions that are often asked by women choosing reconstruction:

- **What if there is cancer in the other breast – wouldn't I be better off having both removed and reconstructed?**
  This is a very common and understandable reaction to the bad news you've just heard. The chances of you having cancer in your other breast are extremely small. Only one out of 200 women who have had breast cancer will develop a new cancer in each subsequent year, and your mammogram will nearly always find any problems. So unless you have other reasons which build up the risk to your other breast in the future (such as a very strong family history), having a double mastectomy is a very big thing to go through without an enormous amount of benefit to you.

- **What size do you want to be?**
  This is an important question to ask yourself, as well as your surgeon, because now is the time when it may be possible to make a change and it may make the results of your surgery much better in the long term. If you are very large with a heavy droopy breast, it can be difficult and sometimes impossible to reconstruct a new breast to match the other side. So it is often a good idea to reconstruct a smaller breast, and then reduce your other side to match. This is usually done a few months later when your reconstruction has settled

down. On the other hand, if you have a small or very small breast, then it's really quite difficult to reconstruct a very small new breast to replace it. The surgeon can often get a much better result by rebuilding a new breast that is bigger than before. This means that the size of your other breast has to be increased to match – and this is often done at the same time. Both of these approaches – building a smaller or larger breast – mean having surgery on both sides. This shouldn't affect the examination of your remaining breast, but it does mean more surgery. It will also give you the best result you can have in the long run. Many questions about surgery on your other breast are answered on p. 128.

Is my surgeon experienced?

This is a really important question and often the most difficult one to ask. After all, you're relying on your surgeon to look after you, and to give you support and advice. And then you find yourself questioning his or her experience at a time when you feel you really need support and advice from the whole breast team. Don't worry about asking this question. Any experienced surgeon won't mind. On the contrary, your surgeon will be happy to tell you about their experience. If they are not experienced, now is the time to find out and to seek advice and treatment elsewhere.

Here's a short list of questions to help you find out more about the experience of your team in breast reconstruction:

- Ask how many reconstructions the team does every year. They should carry out at least twenty to twenty-five cases every year to give them enough experience.

- Does the team do all kinds of reconstruction – subpectoral, latissimus dorsi and autologous reconstruction?

- If not, will they refer you to a unit that does?

- Ask to see all the publications and articles on reconstruction produced by the unit.

- Ask if it is possible to speak to patients treated by the unit and look at written information and pictures of patients.

- Look your surgeon up on the Internet. This will tell you about his or her area of experience, as well as whether they have kept up-to-date.

- Talk to your GP about the kind of services offered by the Breast Unit.

Modern training programmes for breast surgery now include training in breast reconstruction. So there is an increasing chance there will be a surgeon on your team who will be able to carry out your reconstruction and give you all the choices that you need.

Finally, remember that the service is geared around you as a patient, and those treating you will respect your own views and choices. You owe it to yourself to examine all your options and to ask lots of questions. You won't be ready to go ahead until you feel that all your questions have been answered and you've had a good chance to make up your mind.

3

Subpectoral reconstruction and implants

- **Subpectoral reconstruction is the simplest procedure.**
- **Silicone breast implants are safe and are used worldwide.**
- **There are many different shapes and sizes of implants to choose from.**
- **Tissue expanders are adjustable implants.**
- **They may need to be exchanged or removed if they wear out or cause complications.**
- **Recovery takes about four weeks.**

Subpectoral reconstruction

So we're into technicalities already! 'Subpectoral' simply means 'under the pectoralis major muscle' and refers to the surgical technique of creating a pocket underneath the large, fleshy triangular muscle in the upper chest, the pectoralis major (which body-builders refer to as 'pecs') under which a breast implant can be placed. This muscle lies underneath the breast, and there is one on each side of the chest. After mastectomy, an implant placed under the muscle recreates the fullness and volume of the missing breast. This means that the implant is covered by the pectoralis muscle, as well as the overlying skin and fatty tissue. It's the simplest type of reconstruction because your surgeon doesn't have to borrow tissue from another part of the body to rebuild your breast. Because of this, you're more likely to have a shorter hospital stay, a quicker recovery and a smaller chance of complications.We'll come back to the anatomy and the surgical details later, but perhaps we should start by talking about breast implants.

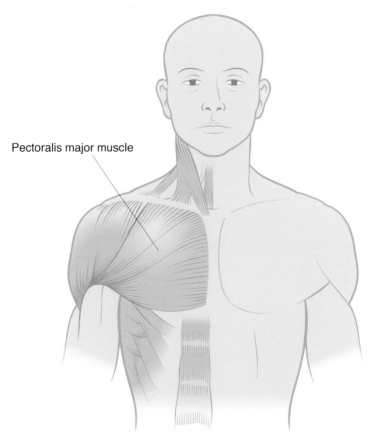

Pectoralis major muscle

The pectoralis major and some other muscles on the front of the chest

Breast implants

Cosmetic breast implants and reconstruction: What's the difference?

There have been so many programmes about cosmetic surgery on television recently that most women will already know about the use of breast implants to increase breast volume and enhance the bust. Celebrity magazines constantly speculate about who might have had a 'boob job' (which in surgical terms is called an augmentation mammoplasty).

The difference between a purely cosmetic augmentation and a breast reconstruction is that after a mastectomy or a major removal of breast tissue there may be nothing left of the original breast. Your surgeon has to recreate not only the volume of the missing tissue, but also has to make sure that there's enough skin and soft tissue to cover the new breast so that it has a natural contour and appearance.

The aim of all breast reconstructions is to create a new breast that looks and feels as normal as possible, and matches your natural, remaining breast. After all, your new breast is one of a pair, but as with all reconstructive techniques sometimes it's also necessary to also work on the opposite side to get the very best symmetry.

Breast implant materials

Any material that is implanted into living tissue has to be well tolerated. Early attempts to increase breast size surgically used a variety of substances with relatively little long-term success. In 1963 two American surgeons introduced the silicone gel implant, which was followed in 1964 by a saline-filled implant. These have been the basis of all breast implants since then, with constant technological developments to improve long-term durability and to make the implants better tolerated in living tissue. All current breast implants are based on the same basic design and use silicone components.

Silicone versus silicon

'Silicone' shouldn't be confused with 'silicon', which is a chemical element. 'Silicon' is the second most common material in the earth's crust and is a component of glass, cement and ceramics. 'Silicones' are synthetic materials, built around a frame of silicon and oxygen atoms. The more the chemical groups are cross-connected (polymerisation), the firmer the consistency of the material. The basic component of breast implant materials is PDMS, or polydimethylsiloxane. This varies in consistency from its softest liquid form, through to gel, then to a firm rubber-like texture, and eventually to a hard material similar to plastic.

Liquid silicones are used as medical lubricants: they are the clear material used to 'grease' the inside of syringes to allow the plungers to move smoothly, and to coat needles so that they can glide into tissue without friction. The 'inertness' of silicones has led to their widespread use for medical applications, and particularly for implanted devices, such as tubing in neurosurgery for draining 'water on the brain', and in cardiac surgery to insulate pacemaker wires. Silicones are also used for artificial joints in the hands and for a whole range of implants, including of course, cosmetic and reconstructive breast implants.

Are silicones safe?

Silicones are very much a part of everyday life. They're added to infant feeding formulas to counteract burping. Babies' dummies are coated with silicone, and it's found naturally in cows' milk. Silicones are also used in the kitchen to coat baking paper to make it non-stick. They're present in processed and manufactured foods, and medicines, such as preparations for infantile colic. Silicone sealants have widespread uses in the kitchen and bathroom. So even though we may not be aware of their presence, we regularly ingest silicones and come into close contact with them every day in our homes.

Concerns about breast implants

Although numerous scientific studies have given strong reassurance that silicone breast implants are safe, some people still have concerns. It is important that if you're considering a reconstruction technique using implants, you should be well informed so that you can make a comfortable decision.

The silicone controversy

In 1992, the United States Food and Drug Administration (FDA) imposed a virtual 'ban' on the use of silicone gel-filled implants, which despite many years of use, were reclassified as 'experimental'. They could only be used in clinical trials and for reconstruction after mastectomy. The use of saline-filled implants was not affected. There were suggestions that silicone gel-filled breast implants caused disease by stimulating tissue reactions and causing connective tissue diseases such as arthritis.

In the UK, a new body was established in 1993 to review the scientific literature. The Independent Expert Advisory group found no evidence of any link between silicone gel breast implants and diseases such as arthritis. In 1998, a new body, the UK Independent Review Group (IRG), carried out an extensive scientific review of all the available evidence Once again, no conclusive evidence was found that breast implants cause abnormal tissue reactions or arthritis. The extensive scientific review included the results of investigation and monitoring in studies from the 1980s onwards. The IRG reviewed a very wide range of studies, concluding that silicones don't have any long-term harmful effects on your body. No links were found with specific illnesses, joint diseases, diseases of the nervous system, breastfeeding or any toxic reactions. In fact, women with breast implants were found to have a lower incidence of breast cancer than the general population, and breast-screening was possible in women with implants. Local effects, such as capsular contracture (scar tissue forming around the implant) were just like the body's normal reaction to any implanted foreign material, rather than to any unusual toxic reaction. Implant durability, rupture and gel-bleeding (the leakage of silicone gel through an intact shell) were all highlighted.

Silicone gel breast implants continued to be used freely in the UK. The European Union carried out its own scientific studies, and in February 2003 voted to allow continued use of breast implants, but with specific measures in place to support patients, assure quality and encourage ongoing research.

Eventually, the weight of the scientific evidence led the FDA to restore the use of gel-filled implants in the USA in 2005, and Canada followed suit. Remember however, that the use of breast implants for reconstruction after mastectomy has never been affected.

The development of silicone implants

Three 'generations' of implants have been developed over the last 40 years. All have an outer shell, or envelope of silicone elastomer 'silicone rubber', and a filler substance, either silicone gel or saline.

'First generation' devices had a thick, smooth walled silicone outer shell, and were filled with silicone gel. In the mid 1970s, 'second generation' implants were brought in with thin outer shells and more liquid silicone gel fillers, in the misguided belief that scar tissue reaction might be reduced. These devices were fragile and had a high rupture rate, so they were discontinued. From the late 1980s, 'third generation' implants were produced with thicker double or triple shells with chemical barriers to silicone leakage, and a thicker, more viscous 'cohesive' gel filler. External rough surface texturing is now almost universal in Europe. This process makes the surface of the implant rough rather than smooth, and this has been shown to cut down the scar tissue reaction around the implant (capsular contracture). Over the last 20 years, 'third generation' implants have been shown to have excellent durability.

Specialised breast reconstruction implants

The cosmetic procedure to increase breast size by using a breast implant is known as augmentation mammaplasty. Your breast size is increased by the insertion of an implant in a surgically created pocket, either directly under your breast tissue (subglandular), or under your pectoralis major muscle – the subpectoral, or submuscular plane, as mentioned on p. 29.

One reason for choosing a deeper tissue plane, and going underneath the muscle, is that some patients who want breast enlargement have very little tissue of their own, so an implant placed under their existing breast tissue would have very little tissue to provide a cushion over the implant. Going more deeply, under the pectoralis muscle, gives the implant an added thickness of soft tissue cover, which is a benefit when patients are very thin or have very little breast tissue of their own to cover the implant.

When a patient comes for a delayed reconstruction after mastectomy, there is no breast tissue left. Skin will also have been removed, leaving a scarred, smooth surface on the chest wall in the place of the breast. The scarred skin lies immediately on top of muscle with no intervening thickness of soft breast tissue. The surgeon needs to recreate not only the volume and fullness of your missing breast, but has also to make sure that there's enough overlying skin to cover your reconstructed breast mound so that it looks natural in terms of softness, with enough 'ptosis' (drooping) to match the shape and contour of your remaining breast.

What are the cosmetic goals of breast reconstruction surgery? Try to imagine a normal female profile, what a woman with a normal body build and proportionate breasts sees when she looks at herself sideways on in the mirror. She sees a natural profile and contour, and soft tissues which droop naturally under gravity, and move on the chest as she turns. After mastectomy, in the absence of adequate skin, simply putting a breast implant under very tight and thin scarred skin would be as if a man had stuffed a large apple into the breast pocket of his shirt. The tight fabric would hold the apple firmly, causing it to jut out, and of course the profile would be nothing like that of a normal female breast.

If an immediate reconstruction is being considered (i.e. in the same operative procedure, immediately after completion of the mastectomy), there'll be more skin available for use in your reconstruction, because a 'skin-sparing' procedure will have removed only your breast tissue, with your skin being preserved to provide cover for your new breast.

Tissue expanders and expander/implants

What is skin or muscle 'expansion'?

If reconstruction is delayed until the mastectomy site has healed (delayed reconstruction), there won't be enough skin left to cover the additional volume of a reconstructed breast. If the reconstructive surgery is carried out immediately after a mastectomy in which both breast and breast skin have been removed (in other words the skin has not been spared), the situation is the same. Even if the skin has been spared, there's a large empty space that the removed breast occupied, and this needs to be filled.

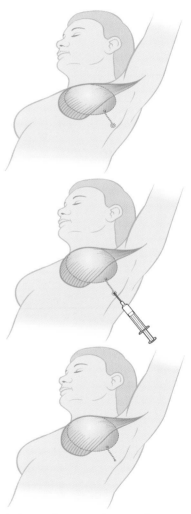

In these situations, the implant is placed under your muscle ('subpectorally'), and the thick layer of muscle needs to be stretched out to fill the empty pocket of skin, pushing your muscle out in a dome shape so that it becomes thin and supple and lies snugly in contact with your overlying skin. The moulding of the soft tissues to form the most naturally shaped breast is achieved with an 'expander' – an expandable bag that can be gradually increased in size to make the surrounding tissues stretch out.

The surgical technique of 'skin expansion' takes advantage of the elasticity of living tissues. If they are gradually stretched, they can expand massively. Think of what happens when a slim woman becomes pregnant: towards the end of pregnancy her abdominal wall is stretched to accommodate the baby. Of course she hopes that as soon as the baby is born, her tissues will tighten again so that she has a taut and firm abdominal wall.

Submuscular expansion stretches the muscle into a dome shape as the expander enlarges

If the period of stretching is relatively brief, and if the stretching has been moderate, there's a much better chance that nature will restore a flat tummy. If, however, there has been a marked increase in weight, and if the baby has been very large (or perhaps there may have been twins or triplets), it's less likely that her abdominal wall will go back to being exactly as it was before. The soft tissues may then be lax with some baggy skin being left.

Actually, this is what skin expansion in breast reconstruction tries to achieve: a permanent excess of tissue to contribute to an ordinary amount of drooping, with the breast implant lying comfortably in a large enough pocket of muscle and skin to move naturally with the body.

Temporary expanders

A temporary expander is an implant made of silicone. It has an empty chamber that can be enlarged by filling it with increasing volumes of fluid. The expander can be inserted at the same time as your mastectomy, or later, as a delayed reconstruction. There will normally be only one scar. Two separate surgical procedures are needed, each under general anaesthetic: the first to place your expander, and the second to remove it once there is a big enough pocket, and to replace it with an implant. Your recovery time after each procedure is about two or three days.

The expander is inserted underneath the soft tissues of your chest wall into the same space that was occupied by your breast. Depending on the design of the implant, a tiny valve may be placed in a separate pocket under your skin near to the expander, to which it is connected by a tube. Saline (sterile salt solution, with the same sodium concentration as body fluids) is injected through your skin into the valve, and passes into the expander. With increasing volumes of saline within your expander, your soft tissues stretch out, and the expansion process continues until your newly created breast is slightly larger than the intended final size. There is an uncomfortable feeling of pressure as the saline goes into the implant, which most women find they can cope with. When the tissues stretch, the feeling of tightness reduces.

At the end of the expansion process, your expander is removed, and it's replaced with a silicone breast implant that will stay in place permanently, to be your definitive breast.

The permanent expander implant

This design of device combines the two different stages of implant reconstruction (expansion and the permanent implant) into a single double-chambered implant. Permanent expanders are available in a range of sizes and shapes. The outer layer contains silicone gel, which gives the implant a more natural feel. The inner layer is an inflatable chamber, which functions as the expander, being stretched with saline injected through the valve.

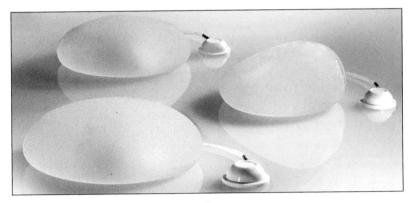

Different shapes of permanent expanders

Blue dye has been put into the inner chamber (the clear space around is the gel-filled outer chamber)

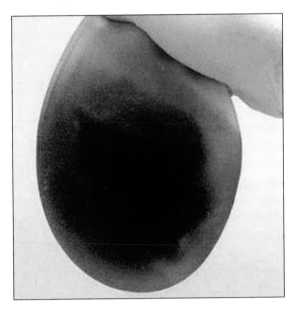

Some designs of permanent expander have a valve that is incorporated into the wall of the device, being part of its permanent structure. Other permanent expanders have an ingenious pull-out system to allow the valve and tube assembly to be removed at the completion of the process, leaving the two-chambered implant in place, at the chosen final volume, as the permanent replacement for the breast. So with this type of permanent expander, when you and your surgeon are happy a simple procedure under local anaesthetic allows the injection valve and tube to be removed. An inner valve seals as the tubing slips out. With a permanent expander implant, you only have to undergo one inpatient operation for the insertion of the implant, with the final valve removal often being a walk-in/walk-out outpatient procedure.

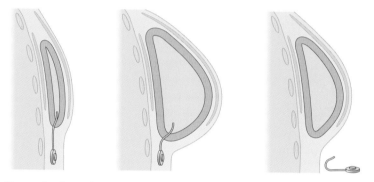

Expander insertion, overexpansion and deflation, and replacement with a permanent implant

What is 'overexpansion'?

Both temporary and permanent expanders can be filled gradually with saline, adding more volume as stretching occurs. However, many surgeons favour the technique of immediate overexpansion, which is suitable for some designs of implant, and is particularly appropriate for delayed reconstructions.

The breast implant is inflated immediately to 80–90% of its intended final overexpanded volume. Of course this can be very uncomfortable, so pain control and sedation are important. However, the expansion process is shortened, and the need for many more injections for gradual stretching may be avoided.

The aim of overexpansion is to create additional skin to contribute to a normal contour, with the implant lying loosely within a mobile soft tissue envelope. However, some other designs of permanent expander incorporate a firmer structured implant which gives its shape to the overlying tissue, so that there is less need to overexpand in order to generate skin.

Bilateral implant reconstruction

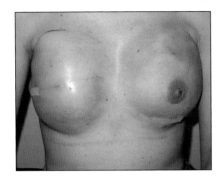 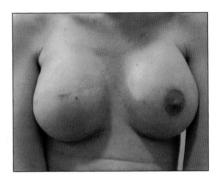

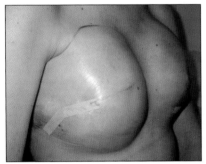 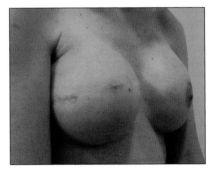

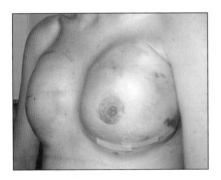 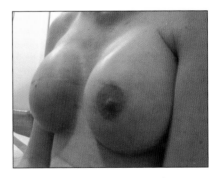

An early postoperative picture showing a delayed reconstruction on the patient's right side, and a subcutaneous (skin-sparing) mastectomy and immediate reconstruction on the left side, using a Becker 'permanent expander' (there is a degree of immediate overexpansion)

The same patient at the completion of implant/expander reconstruction: the overexpansion has been reduced, and final shape and volume have been achieved to her satisfaction

The operation
How will it be for me?

- **Pain**

  At the very least, you should be prepared to feel uncomfortable immediately after the operation and for several days afterwards. Every woman's skin is as different as her pain threshold, so no one can predict exactly how it will be for you. So it's as well to be prepared for the worst. Whilst everyone feels pressure, for some patients the sensation is extremely painful and it may feel difficult to breathe. The discomfort settles as the tissues stretch, but for some women, the tightness and aching may last for several weeks.

- **The valve**

  The valve (if it's part of the structure of the device), will be placed in a separate pocket under your skin, a little way from the implant. You'll be conscious of a bump which you'll be able to see and feel, just under the skin. The valve position is usually on the side of your chest wall, above your bra strap, but your surgeon will choose what's the most appropriate position, bearing in mind the need to balance easy access for injection, whilst avoiding rubbing and chafing where possible. Most women are conscious of the valve being present, and for the vast majority there's no more than mild discomfort. The initial pain of the surgery usually settles over a period of a week or two.

- **Stitches**

  Many surgical wounds are closed with dissolving buried sutures, so there may well be no stitches to remove. When implant reconstruction is undertaken together with a tissue flap (see p. 45), the soft tissues may be inset into the chest wall with stitches, or with surgical staples. These are easily removed and do not cause stitch marks.

- **Drains**

  After fairly extensive surgery, there is inevitably a large raw area in the surgical site which will go on to heal. Great care will have been taken during the operation to detect and seal off any bleeding points, but there's still the risk of oozing from the cut tissue surfaces. Fine tubes are left in the wound, attached to vacuum bottles, to draw off blood and other fluid. When drainage lessens, the drains are removed, about 15 cm of fine tubing being pulled out. There can be a twinge of pain momentarily, and analgesic (pain-relieving) medication is often given before the drains are removed.

- **Going home**
After surgery, you'll need to take things easy for a couple of weeks. You should avoid any activity which causes the muscle to contract. Some everyday tasks, such as lifting a filled kettle, may be surprisingly painful. Plan to have help with everyday activities for a fortnight, but you'll gradually be able to do more and more as the tissues settle and the postoperative discomfort lessens. You shouldn't plan to resume upper body exercises in the gym for perhaps four weeks, and you should make sure that you don't undertake any exercises that stress the chest – press-ups, for example. Lower body exercises will be possible earlier, but make sure that you have good support, for example, wearing a good sports bra under a firm supportive top when running.

Implant reconstruction: Is it right for me?

Advantages of implant breast reconstruction

- Implant surgery, when it's considered feasible, is the simplest surgical technique to achieve a reconstruction. Your surgeon will advise you of any contraindications which would be likely to prevent an implant reconstruction. There aren't any additional scars created elsewhere on the body, and on the chest wall only the original surgical scars are used. Of course implants can be used in conjunction with skin and muscle flaps, and these will entail additional scars (see p. 78). It's very straightforward to replace implants with fresh ones, should the need arise.

Disadvantages and complications of implant breast reconstruction

- **The surgery**
Your operation may be an extensive procedure, particularly if your mastectomy and reconstruction are carried out at the same time. All surgical procedures are associated with the early risks of infection and bleeding, and there will be scarring as the wounds heal. You will stay in hospital under close observation until the risks have reduced

and it's safe to let you go home. A haematoma is a collection of blood within the wound, and whilst drains will prevent collections of blood occurring in most cases, it will occasionally be necessary to return to the operating theatre to remove blood if it collects within the wound and around the implant. After initial healing, scars undergo a gradual process of 'maturation'. Initially, as healing is very active, scars can be raised, red and lumpy. There may be itching and irritation. Over a period of months, scars will soften, flatten and start to blend in with the adjacent tissue. Scarring is of course a part of any surgical procedure, and the final quality of the scar depends as much on the way that you heal as the surgery.

● **Being temporarily lopsided**
During the period of several months when the tissues are being stretched, you may not have a symmetrical bust. Scarves and loose clothing can help to disguise a difference in breast size. However, most women who have been through the expansion process report that other people are not as aware of your appearance as you might think.

● **Capsular contracture**
Your new breast will take its final shape and volume from the breast implant, but clearly this can never become a living part of your body, as happens when soft tissue from the buttock or abdomen is used to make the breast (see p. 72). The implant is foreign to the body and there will always be an interface between the implant and your own tissue. Sometimes there can be a reaction around the implant which can then be distorted by encircling scar tissue. If this is hard and fibrous, it can squeeze the implant and affect its shape and softness. This 'capsular contracture' affects a proportion of women, both after cosmetic implants and after breast reconstruction.

● **Silicone bleeding**
Small amounts of silicone can escape from an intact implant, which does not change shape or lose its structural integrity. This is called silicone bleeding, and minute amounts of silicone can find their way into lymph nodes. They don't cause disease, and of course your lymph nodes will be checked regularly as part of the follow-up for the breast cancer. It's usually very straightforward to distinguish between lymph node enlargement due to a reaction to silicone or caused by breast disease. Scans and needle biopsy may be undertaken by your surgeon to clarify the situation.

● **Implant rupture**

If an implant 'fails', meaning that it leaks or ruptures, it's held within the fibrous capsule and a change in shape or volume may only be slowly apparent. Be assured that extensive scientific studies have shown that silicone gel leaking from cosmetic or reconstructive implants doesn't cause disease, other than a tissue reaction to foreign material.

● **The longer term**

How long do implants last? It's hard to be precise in answering this as there are many different designs of expanders and implants. Anything that is synthetic may wear out, though current implants are engineered to very exacting standards to be as durable as possible over many years.

After your operation

Your other breast

After your implant reconstruction, you'll be followed up until surgery is completed on the reconstructed side. As with other breast reconstruction techniques, it's often helpful to consider surgery to the other breast to gain the best match in size and shape. An over-large breast can be reduced in size (breast reduction), an excessively droopy breast can be uplifted (mastopexy), and a very small breast can be enlarged (augmentation), using the same techniques as used in purely cosmetic surgery (see pp. 130–136).

Your reconstructed breast will need to match your other side in shape and volume, and implants with valves have the advantage that they are very easy to enlarge or reduce in volume. Finally, you may want to have a new nipple and areola created: there are specific surgical techniques for this, with tattooing to restore colour match. These techniques can be applied to all forms of breast reconstruction surgery. Many women are, however, content just to have a nicely matching breast in a bra, even if the breasts are not an exact match in the nude. There is no need for you to have any more surgery once you are content with the way you look. Some women are happy to look normal in clothing, whilst some others do want to sunbathe topless, and happily, surgery can offer reconstructive procedures across the whole spectrum of patients' wishes.

Follow-up

Follow-up visits will continue after completion of all surgical procedures. They give your surgeon the opportunity to ensure that all is well after your breast cancer treatment, and also with the reconstruction. These check-ups are also a regular opportunity to make sure that the implant used in your reconstruction remains problem free. As well as clinical examination, which is adequate in the vast majority of patients, the integrity of the implant can also be confirmed by scans and x-rays if there are any concerns.

> I was 62 and it was nearly 11 years since my mastectomy. I asked the Breast Care Sister whether it was too late to have reconstruction and she thought not. I saw the surgeon and he asked me why I wanted reconstruction. It was really the fact that I had gone from an ordinary prosthesis to a self-adhesive one, which had made me feel much more whole and natural. Having had to give that up, reconstruction presented itself to me as a good option. As I was small, it was suggested that I should have just a tissue expander, rather than anything more major. I was pleased about that.
>
> Preparation for the operation was easy because it was my choice and there was none of the worry of the mastectomy or whether the cancer had spread. I felt more buoyant to cope with it than people who were having first time round operations.
>
> After the operation, it was a bit sore but I only had the painkillers for a couple of days. After that, it was only uncomfortable if I moved. I got up and around the day after the operation and was in hospital for four days. The breast was covered and quite bruised. I looked at it when the dressings were taken off and was very pleased with it because it had been done through the same scar. I had been told what it would look like and that it would take two or more months to settle down, so I wasn't anxiously expecting results at that time.
>
> Because I was 62 and the other breast had lost condition, the surgeon operated on it at the same time, lifting it to match the reconstructed one. It did mean that I had twinges in both breasts at once but that was quite acceptable and also saved another operation.

When I went home, I could do light duties and it was about three weeks before I drove again. It was a month or two before I could do what I wanted in the garden.

The tissue expansion was no problem. It felt a bit tight after each time but I didn't need painkillers. The expanded breast came higher up the chest than I would have liked and to get better parity with the other breast, we had to try inflating and deflating it a couple of times. It is still slightly smaller than the other one because to fill it sufficiently would have caused an imbalance higher up the chest. I am quite happy with it.

"

"
I chose to have a mastectomy, rather than lumpectomy and radiotherapy. Immediate breast reconstruction was not offered in 1988. My lifeline after the mastectomy was knowing that I was going to have a reconstruction. I had been widowed five years before that and there was a new male friend on the horizon. I thought that starting a new relationship might be the time to go for reconstruction. I have always been big-breasted and I wanted a big reconstruction. I wanted to look the same as I had done before.

The reconstruction was not as uncomfortable as I had thought it would be. The worst thing about it was the pressure on my chest, particularly at night. I felt as though I was struggling to breathe because of it. I was told that as time goes by, gravity helps and it is better to stand or sit up rather than lie down. I had to do quite a lot for myself when I got home but I did have some help.

The tissue expansion was done every two weeks. It took ten days after each expansion for the breast to feel reasonable again and then they would add more saline. It was a long and gradual process. The pressure on the chest was uncomfortable and it did help to see someone else who had had it. She was able to tell me that the pressure would pass. The process of expansion took nine months altogether. It is important to allow adequate time and then you can feel confident and put your life together again.

I had to cope with the difference in size between both breasts for a few months. I either wore a scarf, or edge-to-edge jackets, without buttons. The size difference spoils the line of buttoned jackets. If you wear anything with a horizontal line, your eye is drawn to it. I also wore a little bit more make-up to take the eye away from my breasts.

I have the same tissue expander that was inserted in 1988 and the reconstruction is nearly as soft as it was originally. I have good skin sensation, although there is no sensation or erection in the nipple. I find lifting a weight above my head or using a hand-whisk with constant repetition difficult but apart from those two things, I can do everything that I want to.

I am very glad that I had the reconstruction done. Although I did not have a choice of which type, I am perfectly happy with it. It made it easier for me in my relationship. I wanted to make the best of myself and it gave me confidence. I definitely turned the corner psychologically when the reconstruction started. It is in your hands to make the most of life. If reconstruction is part of that, go for it but think carefully about it first.

"

"
I didn't cope very well with the mastectomy and prosthesis but part of that may have been because I knew that I was going to have a breast reconstruction. I was 51 at the time. Immediate breast reconstruction was not available.

I was offered a tissue expander for breast reconstruction. It was very helpful to meet someone who had had one before me. She showed me hers and told me quite a lot about it. The decision to have breast reconstruction has to be the person's own decision. It is very useful to know how long the whole process is going to take.

Afterwards, there was a very tight sensation across my chest and it felt very heavy and hard at first. The drains were taken out and I left hospital after five days.

At home, I wasn't really restricted too much. I didn't do housework and took things easily. I went back to work part-time after four weeks and was full-time after three or four months.

My expander was fully expanded at surgery and then adjusted later. This was started after three months and was very gradual. At that time, the breast was large and quite high up on my chest. I felt quite good about that because I had always wanted to be larger. I bought a big bra and put the comfy that I had after the mastectomy into the other side to even it out. I always wore loose tops and it didn't really show. The whole process of stretching and deflating took a year. I was left the size that I am now for the last month to see that I was happy with it before they took the injection port out. I did find the injection port uncomfortable sometimes. The final match was very good and I was pleased with it.

The reconstructed breast is quite firm and if I am undressed, my natural breast is slightly lower. It is fine in a bra. I can wear any type of bra. I wouldn't hesitate to change in a communal changing room now.

I think that I had the best type of reconstruction for me because I don't take anaesthetics well and don't think that I could have coped with the other options. Mine was probably the easiest option.

I was 46 when it was recommended that I should have bilateral mastectomies. I did not have the option of immediate breast reconstruction, although it was being done at other hospitals.

I got through the mastectomies quite well physically and did the Run for Life five months afterwards. However, I hated the prostheses. I had been quite a large cup size before the surgery but because I had both breasts removed chose to have much smaller prostheses. I didn't want to draw attention to myself any more. The crunch came when we were on holiday in Crete. It was hot and I got fed up with the prostheses, particularly in the swimming pool. It affected my confidence and I decided that I didn't want to go through that again.

I saw a plastic surgeon about breast reconstruction and agonised about the choices but didn't really have a lot of information. He only suggested that I should have a Becker tissue expander. I felt that I wanted to keep the surgery to a minimum, so came to terms with his suggestion.

In retrospect, I think that I would have liked to have seen people who had the other reconstructive operations as well. Recently, three of us who had had different reconstructions were showing another lady who was deciding, and when I saw the other options, they looked better than mine. They had all recovered so well from their more complicated operations and their breasts looked so natural.

Initially, the reconstruction felt very painful. I don't think that I had expected that and should have taken the painkillers on offer. Because the expander had been almost fully expanded before it was put in, I felt as though I had a concrete block sitting on my chest. I had two lots of drains and they were manageable. I went home after a few days.

When I first looked at my new breasts, they looked as I had expected for that stage. They were very high, large and solid. I found that it took me longer to get over the reconstruction than it did for the mastectomy. Getting some arm movements back was a gradual process.

After six months, I had to have the muscle around one implant cut to release a capsule that had formed and that worked.

With tissue expansion, I was a funny shape for some time during the expansion and it was lucky for me that it happened over the winter because I could disguise it with baggy clothes. If it is possible to choose the time, it's worth opting for winter when it is not so hot and uncomfortable.

I used to do a lot of gardening but am still careful with what I do. I am so pleased that I had the reconstruction, regardless of this.

I think that the breasts have become softer in the three years since the operation and one side has changed shape slightly. I wear really soft underwired bras. The reconstructions are quite flat and don't droop, so I can't fill out some bras. Other types of reconstructions seem more natural. It was very difficult with clothes before reconstruction. I still find some hard but am more confident now.

It may be easier to accept mastectomies and reconstructions when both sides are involved because I have nothing left to remind me of what I had. It was traumatic at the time but easier later. The reconstructions have given me so much confidence, which I didn't think I would get back after the mastectomies. Even if there are a few drawbacks at the time of surgery, reconstruction changes your attitude to everything.

Because of the type of cancer that I had and the risk of recurrence in the other breast, I was offered the jackpot of double mastectomies and breast reconstruction. My treatment until then had been long-winded and I decided to have this to get it over and done with. Because I had lost a lot of weight after chemotherapy, they could not use the tummy muscle. I had no tummy and even less on my back. It was recommended that I had tissue expanders for the reconstruction.

I found the surgery very painful. The first set of implants was very painful, so they were swapped for something softer. I think that things might have felt tight because I am so slim.

As far as the shape of the reconstructions is concerned, if anything, there has been a slight drooping of the breasts. The tightness has always been there. The breasts match quite well because they were done at the same time.

The main thing that I would advise others is to get help for tightness, if it occurs, as soon as possible, rather than think that it will go away. My friends who have had breast reconstruction did not find it painful. They are all larger breasted and this makes quite a difference.

I am glad that I had the reconstructions because they have given me shape. I don't have to worry or feel embarrassed in shops or on a hot day.

4 Reconstruction with latissimus dorsi (LD) flap

- **LD reconstruction is a very reliable and popular technique.**
- **It can sometimes be done without using an implant or expander.**
- **It's used for both immediate and for delayed breast reconstruction.**
- **Your reconstructed breast will look and feel very natural.**
- **It requires major surgery.**
- **Recovery takes about six to eight weeks.**

Using live tissue from another part of your body to reconstruct your breast has been a major new development in breast reconstruction over the last twenty years. In fact, it's quite remarkable that tissue will heal into place when it's been moved from one part of your body to another. Most tissue that can be moved like this is made from muscle, fatty tissue and skin, and these structures are called myocutaneous flaps. The use of living tissue to reconstruct a lost breast is a major advance. The new breast is made of soft, warm, living tissue, which can be shaped to look like your original breast.

Two different approaches are used by surgeons to make sure a myocutaneous flap has a good enough blood supply to remain healthy and to heal into place once it's been moved. The first approach is to leave the flap attached to its blood supply or 'pedicle'. The pedicle is rather like an umbilical cord, with the 'mother's end' of the pedicle remaining attached to the place where the flap tissue was taken from – the 'donor site'. The second approach is to divide the pedicle or umbilical cord before removing the flap to its new position. This is called a 'free' flap, because it's been freed from its own blood supply. The surgeon then has to use a highly specialised technique to join the blood vessels in the pedicle to the blood vessels in the region of the mastectomy. The vessels are so small that this needs to be done using a microscope, so the other name for this procedure is a 'free tissue transfer' or a 'microvascular flap'.

The best donor site is one where the loss of donor tissue doesn't disfigure the area where the tissue is taken from. The two commonest donor sites are on the back and on the abdomen. The LD flap is taken from the back and is discussed in this section. The transverse rectus abdominus myocutaneous (TRAM) flap is taken from the abdomen and is discussed in the next section.

Implant-based LD reconstruction

One of the most popular and widely used types of breast reconstruction in the UK today is a technique using both the LD flap and an implant or expander. This is because it's a very reliable and adaptable technique that can give consistently good results for a wide range of women. Some aspects of implant-based LD reconstruction are very similar to auto-logous LD flap reconstruction but there are some important differences. This information in this section will help you to understand the differences so that you and your surgeon can decide which is the best operation for you. The main difference between the two techniques is that following autologous LD flap reconstruction the whole of your reconstructed breast is made from your own tissues. But after implant-based LD reconstruction, a little less than half of your new breast is made from your own tissues and the rest is made from an implant. This is usually an adjustable implant, called an expander. This means that less tissue needs to be taken from your back to do the reconstruction, but you'll have an implant in your new breast. This often gives your reconstructed breast a very good shape and appearance, which can be adjusted after your operation, but it does mean that there can be some additional complications that you don't get with autologous LD flap reconstruction – and also some that you can avoid.

Deciding if implant-based LD reconstruction is one of your options

Implant-based LD reconstruction is suitable for a wide range of women. This is because the combination of an adjustable expander and a fleshy flap gives your surgeon the opportunity to rebuild a life-like breast of almost any shape or size. Because it's a combination of two different approaches – an implant and a flap – it's got some of the advantages as well as some of the diasadvantages of each approach when used by itself.

66
Having a breast reconstruction at the same time as the mastectomy mattered to me. I am a singer and performer and need to wear suitable clothes. I need to wear low-cut tops and the first gig that I sang in again was two months after the operation. I wasn't worried about my breast, but only that the scar on my back didn't show. I found that the operation had not affected my voice or my confidence at all.

I didn't know anything about breast reconstruction before it was recommended. I was given a lot of information in the clinic and later by the breast care nurse. I found that reading the information was the most helpful. I didn't particularly want to talk to anyone else who had had reconstruction. I knew what the diagnosis was and just wanted to get the operation done.

I was expecting to be in a lot of pain after the operation. In fact, there was a lot of numbness but I have had worse toothache. The only thing that was difficult was sleeping in a comfortable position.

I didn't see my new breast until about six days after the operation, when I was able to have a shower. I looked in a big mirror and it looked great. My partner was amazed at how good it looked and my friends thought that it was fantastic.

By the time that I got home, after ten days, I wasn't restricted very much. Some things were difficult to stretch for initially.
99

So when can it be used to reconstruct your breast? Because it's a combined technique, it can be used in almost all of the situations when either an autologous LD flap or an implant can be used. This means that like autologous LD flaps, it's a good technique for immediate and delayed reconstruction – for women who have their breasts reconstructed either during or after their mastectomy

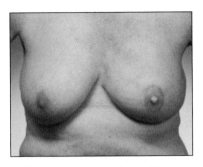 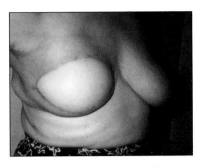

Left mastectomy and immediate implant-based LD flap reconstruction, followed by nipple reconstruction

Delayed implant-based LD flap reconstruction of the right breast

" I knew that I was going to need a mastectomy because the breast cancer involved the nipple. I just thought that the breast had better go, and the sooner the better. My priority was to remove the cancer, get the chemotherapy and radiotherapy out of the way and then when everything was just right, have the reconstruction.

I did not like the real prosthesis after the mastectomy, so wore a softie, which was not sweaty. I did not want to wear the bras that the shop advised, so I wore what I wanted to wear, to be as normal as I could. I went on holiday three weeks after the mastectomy and the swimming helped my arm. I got a suntan and came back feeling good. My children were eight and fifteen at the time and they coped because I was positive. I went back to work during the chemotherapy because it stopped me from sitting at home.

When discussing reconstruction choices, I was attracted to the latissimus dorsi with an implant because I had seen people who had had them before and knew that it would look right for me. It is always worth talking to people who have had reconstruction, to see the finished breast when making up your mind. When I was making the decision, I was on my own. I am now back with my daughter's father.

I had the reconstruction eight months after the last chemotherapy, with radiotherapy in between. The skin had settled down from the radiotherapy by the time that I had the operation. I felt fantastic after the operation and looked at the reconstructed breast straight away. I showed lots of people and was glad that I didn't have to think about a prosthesis again. I threw it away. My arm was fine this time and I didn't need physiotherapy afterwards.

"

"

I was offered a mastectomy and immediate reconstruction but I decided to delay the reconstruction because I felt that if I had to have any treatment afterwards, there was a chance that the new breast might be damaged. I think that I made the right decision.

I went into the choices for reconstruction very thoroughly. I read a bit about it in a book I was given and looked at the websites. I also talked to the breast care nurse in great detail. I was able to see what an implant looked like, as well as being shown photographs. I met someone locally who had reconstruction and couldn't believe it when I saw it. I knew that my reconstruction would not be as good as that because she had hers done at the same time as the mastectomy. I spent a long time weighing up the advantages and disadvantages before I finally said that I would go ahead.

There was only one reconstruction available to me because I had had so many operations on my tummy in the past. Originally, I said that I did not want an implant. I later realised that if I didn't, there was no way that I could have it done. Having taken facts about implants into account, I thought that perhaps it was not such a bad thing after all. It was my decision and no one has tried to influence me. I felt that is right because I didn't want people telling me what I should do. Since the reconstruction, everybody has said that I did the right thing. My husband has been brilliant and has supported me all the time.

"

Like autologous LD flap reconstruction, implant-based LD reconstruction is very useful for women who have badly scarred, thinned or irregular skin around their mastectomy area because of previous surgery, radiotherapy or complications from previous treatment. This is because it 'puts back' tissue which has been lost or damaged, and replaces it with healthy, normal, soft living tissue from your back. It's also very suitable if you're a woman with a more mature breast shape, where most of the volume of your breast lies in the lower part of your breast (or lower 'pole'), below your nipple.

> 66
>
> When being told by the surgeon that I needed a mastectomy, I was asked whether I had thought about breast reconstruction. I discussed the practical aspects and was shown some photographs but didn't ask enough questions, for example how long the operation and recovery would last and how painful it would be. I just assumed that he would reconstruct and that would be that. I was quite naive. I don't think that anything would have put me off because to me having a reconstruction meant that everything would be as normal as possible. Once I had made my decision, I did not sit and worry about it.
>
> I was given the option of speaking to another patient but didn't do it because I had made up my mind. If I had been in two minds, seeing somebody else would have been extremely helpful.
>
> I wasn't expecting the operation to be as painful as it was. Again, it was probably a bit of naivety because I knew that it was a big operation. Also, I had never had serious surgery before. I got up the next day. I needed help and was really surprised how weak I felt. The drips and drains were no problem.
>
> 99

Because it's a good option after previous radiotherapy treatment, implant-based LD reconstruction can also be used if you have to have a mastectomy for a recurrent cancer when your cancer was previously treated by lumpectomy and radiotherapy. And finally, it's often recommended for women who decide to have both breasts removed (bilateral risk-reducing mastectomy) and reconstructed at the same time. This is a major operation that can take four to six hours, even when two teams of surgeons are operating alongside each other. The cosmetic results of this type of surgery are often extremely good because the breasts can be reconstructed to match each other.

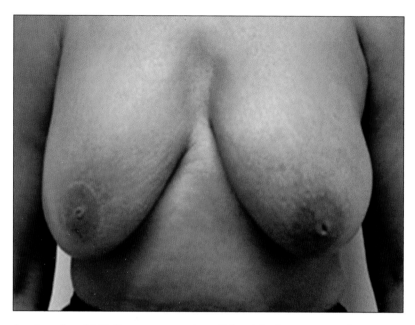

Implant-based LD flap reconstruction of the right breast to match ptosis (or 'droop') of the left breast

66

Three years after I had a lumpectomy, chemotherapy and radiotherapy for breast cancer, I was told that they had found changes on the mammogram and I needed a mastectomy. I was 40 and I was devastated. Life had gone back to normal for me after the lumpectomy.

I did not know anything about mastectomy or reconstruction. I would have walked away from the surgery if I hadn't been convinced that the cancer wouldn't go away on its own. When you are so fit and well, it is hard to believe that you have cancer. Although the reconstruction was only cosmetic, I don't think that I would have been happy without a breast. When I had the lumpectomy, it was just a very small scar. I did have scars from the radiotherapy on my breast. Considering reconstruction on top of that was difficult. I made the decision to have the surgery because of my children, who were nine and twelve years old at the time. You have to do the positive thing and get on with it.

When I first woke up from the operation, I felt that it was behind me and I was on the road to recovery. I had lots of reservations before I looked at the reconstructed breast but I knew that it was going to be all right because I had every confidence in the surgeon.

I could do everything when I went home but it took quite a while to get my strength back. I wouldn't say that it is an easy operation because it was six months before I could sleep on my side. That was a minor thing, though. I had nearly six weeks off work.

I had a nipple reconstructed six months later. I did lead life as normally as possible but nothing was just right until the surgery was finished.

It is four years since the reconstruction and the appearance has changed over the time. The shape has got better, the breast feels softer and it has dropped. The scars on my back are well healed and my breasts match well. There is nothing that I can't do with my arm.

”

When can't this technique be used? There are some definite 'no's' and some 'maybe not's'. It definitely shouldn't be used in women who don't want an implant. And like autologous LD flaps, it can't be used if the blood supply to the muscle has been lost or the muscle itself has been divided and damaged. Moreover, it's best avoided it if you have medical conditions that increase your risks after major surgery. This includes conditions such as heart failure, circulatory problems, lung disease or stroke, or if you're very markedly overweight. It's also important that you're aware if you need radiotherapy after your mastectomy, there's a 50/50 chance that your new breast will become firm and sometimes mis-shapen and uncomfortable.

So if there's a real likelihood of needing radiotherapy, it may be better for you to choose an autologous LD flap or TRAM flap reconstruction, or even delay your reconstruction until you've had your radiotherapy. In the future, new techniques being developed, such as sentinel node biopsy, will be able to help your surgeon to predict if you're going to need to have radiotherapy, so that together you can decide which is the best operation for you.

There is one situation where using LD and an implant is one of the only options. This is in slim women with medium- to large-sized mature-shaped breasts who want a reconstruction that doesn't reduce the size of their new breast, and that looks like their other breast. Because they are slim they don't have enough of their own tissue on their back, on their tummy or even on their buttocks to reconstruct their breast. In this situation, using an implant combined with an LD flap is an ideal solution. This approach is especially suitable if someone like this is requesting reconstruction some time after mastectomy and radiotherapy.

Surgical technique

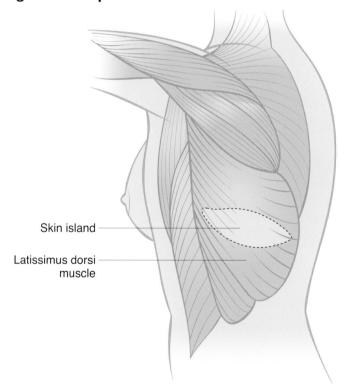

Skin island

Latissimus dorsi muscle

LD anatomy

On your back there are two large triangular muscles – the LD muscles – one on each side. They extend from the tip of your shoulder blade to your spine and down to your hip bone (pelvis). The muscles are attached by a tendon to your upper arm. The blood supply and nerve supply come from the blood vessels in your armpit (axilla) and are usually healthy and working well, even if all the lymph glands in the axilla have been removed. Although the LD muscle lies on your back, it's actually a shoulder muscle and is used to push yourself or pull yourself up – when you're involved in activities such as mountain climbing, rowing, shovelling, cross-country skiing and butterfly-style swimming. Only athletes or competitive golfers will miss the extra strength of this muscle, which is why it's used quite commonly for reconstruction of other defects, such as broken limbs, reanimation of paralysed faces and so on, without interfering with normal day-to-day activities. Other muscles around your shoulder girdle are able to take over the function of the LD and most patients return to their usual work, sporting or leisure activities within three to six months after surgery.

Before your operation, your surgeon will normally ask you what size you'd like your reconstructed breast to be – bigger, smaller or the same? If this isn't mentioned, you should bring it up because now's the time to have this discussion. This will decide what size implant or expander will be used. Also ask your surgeon whether the implant or expander will be shaped – like a teardrop – or will be a rounder type. The shaped type is generally more suitable for the more mature breast shape, and the rounder type for a younger looking, more prominent breast.

Your surgeon should explain to you that with an expander, the 'injection port' – the small chamber that is used for injection of salt water (saline) into your expander after the operation – can be felt under the skin. This is usually felt as a lump, either below the breast or behind the breast, near where the cup of your bra meets your bra strap.

Just before your operation, your surgeon will visit you and draw some lines on your breast or mastectomy region. This is like a 'road map' to make sure that your new breast is in the best possible position. Some lines will also be drawn on your back to help to show exactly how much muscle needs to be 'harvested' for your reconstruction. Your surgeon may also ask you to put on your bra so that your scar can be accurately positioned to be hidden by your bra strap or bikini strap.

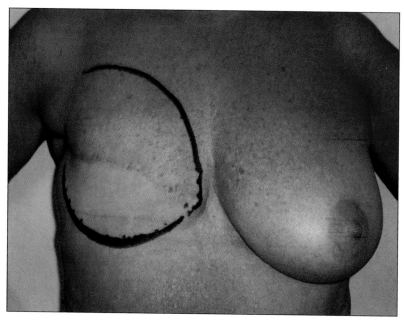

'Mark-up' before implant-based LD reconstruction showing where the new breast will sit on the chest wall

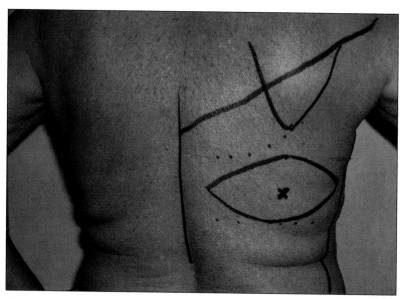

'Mark-up' before implant-based LD reconstruction showing the skin and muscle outline on the back

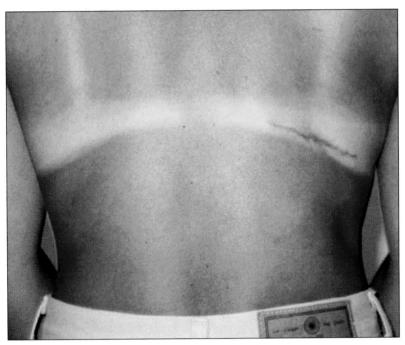

Scar under bra line after implanted-based LD flap reconstruction

The actual operation is very like the operation for autologous LD flap reconstruction. There are a few differences because you're having an expander put in and the flap itself isn't so large and bulky. This means the incision on your back is usually smaller than the one used for autologous LD flap reconstruction. Also, the 'donor site', or space left behind once your muscle has been removed, is smaller. Because of this, the drainage of fluid coming out of a small tube put in this space after your operation is usually less than after an autologous LD flap operation.

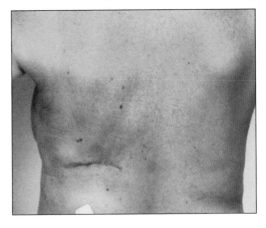

Small scar on the back after implant-based LD reconstruction

66 I was 66 when I was told that I had breast cancer and needed a mastectomy. I was shattered. All my life I had thought that breast cancer was about the worst thing that could happen to me because I would be disfigured. The week before the diagnosis, I saw a film showing breast reconstruction. So my response was 'Please do a reconstruction at the same time.' Anything to help me keep my femininity and be able to present myself to the world as the same person was important.

I was then given plenty of detailed information which only confirmed my decision. It was three weeks before Christmas, so engagements were cancelled and I asked for the operation as soon as possible. The breast care nurse was very helpful and she introduced me to another patient with a similar breast reconstruction. She was lovely and had a list of things that were unexpected when she had her operation. We worked our way through it with a cup of coffee. I would say that people should certainly consider talking to other patients because it is often easier talking to them rather than those close to you. I couldn't talk that way to my daughter because I didn't want to burden her. 99

66 I went home with the drain in and it was manageable. It is easy to catch it on door handles, though. I could do everything. It would not be difficult for someone who lived on their own. I did have to go back as an outpatient and have fluid drained from my back four times but didn't mind because I couldn't feel it. I went to the gym two weeks after the reconstruction and just did leg exercises to begin with. It was several weeks before I did arm exercises. 99

When your 'flap' has been freed up from the surrounding tissues, it's passed around the outside of your chest, through your armpit and into the mastectomy 'pocket' that your surgeon has prepared for it. Up until now, the operation performed by your surgeon is much the same as the operation for an autologous LD flap. The only difference is that the amount of tissue taken from your back is less. From now on the operation's a bit different. Instead of 'modelling' the flap by folding it to make the shape of your new breast, the flap is sewn into the edges of the space that was left behind after the mastectomy. This makes a kind of 'sandwich' of muscles – your LD muscle in front, and your pectoral muscle behind. Your surgeon completes the reconstruction by sliding a deflated expander or an implant in between these two muscles, so that it becomes the 'filler' lying between the two muscle layers of the sandwich.

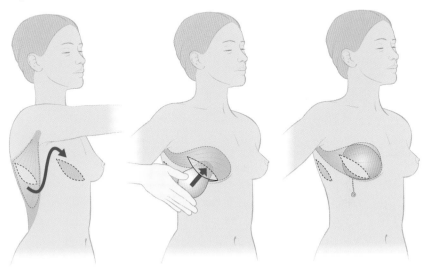

Inserting the expander under the LD flap

If an expander is used, it's now inflated with a solution of saline, so that the size of the new breast is as close as possible to your natural breast. The small injection port is linked to a small tube that is connected to the expander, and the port is positioned in a convenient place under your skin.

Symmetry surgery

Because expanders enable your team to adjust the size of your breast after the operation, fewer women need surgery to adjust the size and shape of their natural breast than after using non-adjustable implants, or after autologous LD reconstruction. If there's still some 'lopsidedness' once expansion has been completed, then a small number of women will opt to have a breast reduction or a mastopexy (see pp. 130–132) to produce a more symmetrical result. It's much better to do this after your reconstruction has settled down, rather than at the time of your reconstructive surgery.

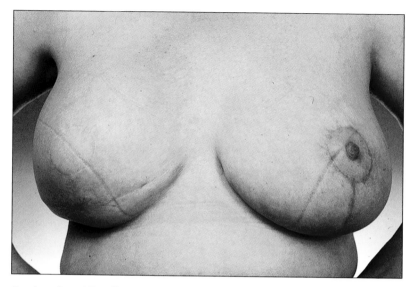

Implant-based LD flap reconstruction of the right breast and reduction of the left breast for symmetry

> 66 I had surgery on my other breast to make it match the reconstruction four months after the mastectomy. The Breast Care Nurse assured me that although it looked very square, the shape would improve in time, and it has. My appearance would have been very odd if I had not had this second operation. The breasts match fairly well. I wear off-the-peg bras but not underwired ones. It is better to have a reconstruction than no breast. I can wear normal clothes and feel normal. I just forget about it. 99

The scale of the operation, success rates and complications

The scale of the operation is very similar to having an autologous LD reconstruction. Although there is a little less surgery to 'harvest' the flap, this is counterbalanced by the extra surgery needed to prepare and position the expander in your new breast. As with the autologous LD, it's a highly reliable flap and it's very rare to have problems with the blood supply. The problems with healing of your mastectomy skin are also much the same, with a higher risk of skin death (known as necrosis) and skin loss in smokers. The problems caused by loss of fatty tissue on the surface of your flap are avoided, because much less fatty tissue is attached to your flap. The wound on your back tends to heal better because it's smaller, and there is less extensive surgery underneath it.

The main difference in complications are linked to the use of implants or expanders. These are avoided with autologous LD flap reconstructions. They aren't very common, and can either happen soon after surgery or later on. Complications soon after surgery include infection and a collection of blood, called haematoma formation. If you get an infection around your implant or expander, it usually means your surgeon will have to remove it. You'll then have to wait for your infection to settle down before it's possible to put it back in again. If you develop bleeding and a haematoma around your implant, this will often settle by itself. If it continues, your surgeon may have to drain the blood and stop the bleeding, but it's not usually necessary to remove the implant in this situation.

Later on, you may develop some thickened scar tissue around your implant or expander, which may make your reconstructed breast look distorted, and feel hard and painful. When this happens, it's possible to cut away the scar tissue, which can cure the problem, but it sometimes returns. In a small number of women, their expanders will rupture, often ten or more years after the initial surgery. When this happens, your surgeon will need to replace it with a new one.

66 I was 67 when I had breast reconstruction. Once the operation was over, I didn't feel too bad. I was walking around the next day and went home after a week. I could do most things at home but tired easily. I couldn't reach high things for the first three weeks. I drove again after six weeks. I don't think that the strength in my arm was affected.

I had to have the fluid drained from my back, where the muscle was moved, for nine weeks as an outpatient. Once that stopped, it was easier to get back to a normal lifestyle.

The reconstructed breast is slightly smaller than my other breast but it doesn't really bother me. I don't think that anybody would notice. I don't have to wear special bras and you don't really see it under clothes.

I am all for going for it anyway. It is a very personal thing. Some
people do have complications and there is always the risk. It was
very helpful having the contact with the breast care nurses and
knowing that I could phone them if I was worried about
anything. I felt I was normal again after having the
reconstruction, it helped psychologically.

"

Advantages of implant-based LD flap reconstruction

This approach is safe, reliable, adaptable and widely available. It's
suitable for a wide range of women with a big range of breast shapes
and sizes. It usually results in smaller scars on the back, which heal
more reliably. The size of the reconstructed breast can be changed
after the operation, and there's less need to alter the normal breast to
make it match the reconstruction.

Disadvantages of implant-based LD flap reconstruction

The main disadvantages with this technique are related to the use of
implants or expanders. The complications are uncommon, and affect
less than 5% of women. If they do happen to you, it may mean that your
implant of expander will have to be removed and replaced at a later date.
If you develop problems with scar tissue, this can usually be corrected
by fairly minor further surgery. In the long run, your implant may need
to be exchanged for a new one if it shows signs of leakage or rupture.
Perhaps the most important disadvantage is the fact that radiotherapy
can undo the good results from this approach. Even autologous LD flap
reconstruction can be adversely affected by radiotherapy, but these
effects are greater when implants or expanders are used.

"
I looked at the breast the first morning because the nurse looked
at it and said that it looked really good. After that, I showed
everyone who came that I knew well. My husband had a quick
glance the first day and his reaction was 'Oh, that's all right isn't
it?' He wouldn't express himself more fully than that. The fact
that I was so positive helped him.

Getting home was difficult. I couldn't get comfortable without
the triangular pillow that I had in hospital. Other than that, I was

fairly OK. I couldn't do very much in the first few days. I just came downstairs and the cat sat on me. I did go with my neighbour to the local shop but I didn't do anything energetic.

Fluid collected on my back where the muscle had been moved for four weeks. It was only a problem in as much as I kept on thinking that it wasn't getting better. I felt better after it had been drained and then it filled up again. I was able to go abroad after four weeks, taking care.

I only had the tissue expansion done a couple of times and it wasn't painful.

"

Autologous LD flap reconstruction

One very popular method has been developed to reconstruct part of a breast or a whole breast using nothing but your own tissues. It's called autologous LD flap reconstruction because it's based on making use of the LD muscle, skin and fatty tissue from the back to rebuild the breast without using an implant.

Deciding if autologous LD flap reconstruction is one of your options

This is a particularly good option for women who want a reconstruction at the time of the mastectomy (immediate reconstruction) and may need radiotherapy after surgery. The autologous LD flap can also be used to rebuild your breast, sometimes months or years after your mastectomy (delayed breast reconstruction), but the amount of spare skin on your back is frequently limited and as a result, the reconstructed breast is often less droopy. An uplift of your opposite breast is therefore required more often than in immediate breast reconstruction, when a much smaller area of breast skin is excised and the original skin 'envelope' is filled with the flap tissues. This technique is also a good alternative for patients who require reconstruction of both breasts either at the same time – in women with cancers in both breasts, or for risk-reducing mastectomy – or as a staged procedure should a second cancer appear in the remaining breast at any time.

" I was really determined that I didn't want to have an implant, so breast reconstruction was narrowed down to two options. The reconstruction using my tummy might have had complications later, so I didn't want that. I am quite active, particularly with gardening. I decided to have an immediate latissimus dorsi reconstruction, using just the back muscle to make the breast. "

Surgical techniques

The LD flap is particularly suited for breast reconstruction because the muscle lies directly underneath your skin. This allows a skin patch (also called a 'skin island') of almost any size and shape to be moved safely together with your muscle and with a layer of fatty tissue on the surface of your muscle to wherever the muscle will reach while it is still attached to its blood supply from the axilla. By taking extra layers of fatty tissue on top, below, above and in the front of the muscle, it's possible to double the volume of the flap and avoid the use of an additional implant for reconstruction of small to moderate-sized breasts.

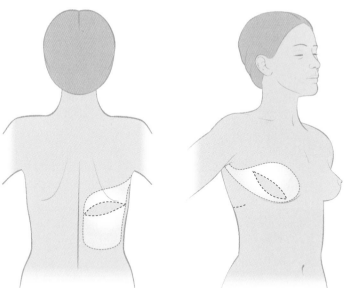

Autologous LD flap reconstruction

The LD muscle, together with the fat and the skin island, are moved through a tunnel under the skin of your armpit, which may have already been created by removal of the glands in this area, to the front of your chest. During your mastectomy, some breast skin, including the skin of the nipple, together with any skin that may be scarred or involved in the cancer and the breast itself will be removed. The skin island from your back can be inserted like a dart into the space surrounded by your remaining breast skin and the muscle and fat can be folded underneath to fill up the space created by your removed breast. This builds up a breast with your own tissues, avoiding the use of a breast implant.

The operation will leave a slightly curved scar on your back, usually at the level of the bra strap and therefore hidden as much as possible. The amount of back skin showing on your reconstructed breast depends on the amount of breast skin that needs to be removed. If you have a delayed breast reconstruction, your surgeon will usually need to take a larger amount of skin from your back than if you have an immediate reconstruction. A reconstruction using LD isn't possible if you have had previous surgery with a scar on the ribcage such as a lung or heart operation. This is because it may have divided the muscle or the blood vessels or nerves that keep this muscle alive (called the neuro-vascular pedicle).

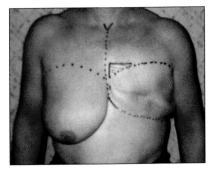 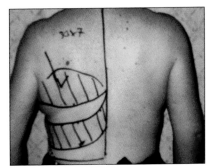

Marking the patient's skin before delayed autologous LD flap reconstruction

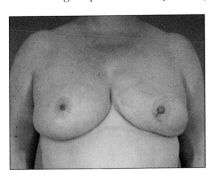 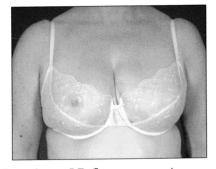

Post-operative pictures following delayed autologous LD flap reconstruction

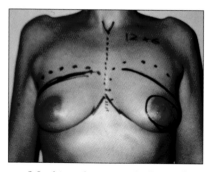 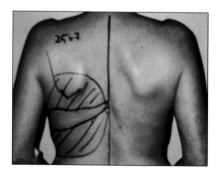

Marking the patient's skin before immediate autologous LD flap reconstruction

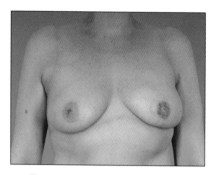 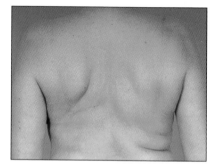

Post-operative pictures following immediate autologous LD flap reconstruction

Symmetry surgery

As with all types of breast reconstruction that use a woman's own tissue, there's a limit on how big a breast can be reconstructed. Surgeons can only take as much tissue as there's available on your back, but most women have enough tissue to reconstruct a breast of average size (B to C cup). If your other breast is very large or very droopy, then there are two options. Your larger breast can be reduced and uplifted to match your reconstructed breast. This would result in two smaller breasts with a more uplifted appearance and may be the preferred option for most women with very large and very droopy breasts. Alternatively, it's possible to increase the size of the smaller, reconstructed breast with a traditional implant or 'lipofilling'. Lipofilling is a special form of 'fat transfer', which moves fatty tissue from other areas of your body into the reconstructed breast to increase the size or even out the irregularities. Breast implants should be avoided in immediate LD reconstruction if there's any real chance that your team will advise you to have postoperative radiotherapy. This is because the chance of hardening of the implant after radiotherapy ('capsular contracture') is very high.

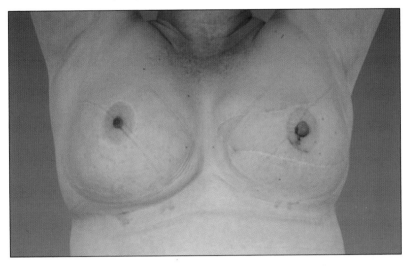

Reconstruction with left autologous LD flap and reduction of the opposite breast to achieve symmetry

> **❝** I had chemotherapy and radiotherapy after the reconstruction and worked during the treatments. My breast doesn't seem to be any different after the radiotherapy.
>
> I went back to wearing underwired bras quickly after the reconstruction.
>
> I would say to someone considering reconstruction to do it. It makes you continue to feel like a woman and you also only have to go through it once. The whole experience has made me think that I should stop and live for today. Obviously we all hope that we won't have to face it but having done so, you have to be as positive as possible. There were days when I thought that it was horrible and didn't know how to go on but I talked myself through it and got on again. You should take the opportunities that you are given so that you come out feeling as complete a woman as you can. **❞**

The scale of the operation, success rates and complications

The LD reconstruction is performed under general anaesthetic and will take your surgeons about four hours for a delayed reconstruction, when the breast has been removed already. An immediate reconstruction will take four hours if there are two teams of surgeons performing the mastectomy and the reconstruction at the same time. When one team of surgeons is performing the whole operation, it takes about five or six hours, as your breast has to be removed first before doing your reconstruction. You'll stay in hospital for about seven days, depending on how much fluid is draining from your wound. Your recovery from surgery will take six to eight weeks. During this time you'll need to have intensive physiotherapy to make sure that your shoulder function returns to normal as quickly as possible.

> After the operation I got up as soon as I could. My back felt very numb. I really didn't have a lot of pain. I just felt a bit wobbly. After about three days, I went for a walk around the hospital. That gave me confidence. I looked at the reconstruction after a couple of days and it wasn't as bad as I thought that it was going to be. The breast was higher up than I had expected and it was bigger because it was swollen from the bruising after the operation. I was in hospital for one week. I didn't do any housework for some time and lifting anything heavy was difficult.
>
> I was given exercises by the physiotherapist in hospital to do at home. I did not realise how important that was. My back became stiff while I was having radiotherapy and I had some more physiotherapy. I wish that I had had more physiotherapy help earlier.
>
> By about nine months, I still couldn't do the things that I loved like swimming and gardening. I found that I couldn't push a full-sized shopping trolley and staying in one position for too long was difficult. Some days I felt quite frustrated and had to be very patient, particularly with the gardening season.
>
> It is now over two years since the reconstruction and I still have some stiffness in my back but it is much improved. I continue

with the exercises and the swimming. I can now do most things in the garden but for shorter periods. I have to change position frequently. I cannot carry as much as I used to but I don't really feel restricted. When it is cold, my back muscles do stiffen up. 99

66 I felt a lot better than I thought I was going to after the operation. I was not in pain as such, it was discomfort. The drains were a little bit daunting and awkward but you adjust and cope with them. I got up and around the next day, as well as starting exercises gradually. My arm was quite stiff but the movement came back fairly quickly.

The scars were very neat and I kept my own skin. I was only missing the nipple.

When I got home, I could do all the normal things but I wasn't allowed to do any heavy lifting for six weeks. My mum came to stay but I did all the washing and things like that. I did my exercises regularly and my arm movement got better.

Some fluid did collect on my back after the drains were taken out. It was drained once, some more collected but it just dissolved back into my body itself.

I drove again after five weeks. I went gently to start with. I had been concerned about having to make any quick movements but that was all right. 99

LD flap breast reconstruction is a very versatile, safe and reliable technique. The overall success rate of the autologous LD flap is more than 99%. Only serious damage to the blood vessels in the armpit that keep the muscle alive (the neuro-vascular pedicle) could cause the flap to die off and fail. Some fatty tissue will be lost in about 14% of women. This happens most commonly in very overweight patients who need reconstruction of very large breasts. Loss of some of the breast skin that has been saved during mastectomy or delayed healing of the back wound happens in 10–15% of cases and it's five times more likely in smokers. The most common problem with the back wound is a collection of wound fluid under the skin, which is called a seroma.

Your surgeon may need to draw off this fluid with a needle and a syringe if it becomes troublesome – sometimes on several occasions until it settles down. The injection of a weak steroid at the first time the fluid is drawn off or the use of special sutures to close off the space during the initial operation will help to reduce the chances of seroma formation.

Advantages of autologous LD flap reconstruction

The LD flap breast reconstruction is a very adaptable, predictable and reliable technique. As with reconstruction using abdominal tissue, it's able to provide a completely natural reconstruction with your own tissues, but it avoids having to take muscle from your abdominal wall. It also avoids the complications of free tissue transfers (see p. 96). This technique is therefore suitable even for patients who have other health problems and may be too high-risk for free tissue transfer.

The biggest advantage of the autologous LD flap is that only your own tissues are used to rebuild your breast. This avoids all the potential complications of breast implants or tissue expanders, such as infection, loss of the implant, capsular contracture and the need for replacement of the implant at a later stage.

This type of reconstruction will also withstand postoperative radiotherapy much better than most other types of breast reconstruction. Because of this, it's well suited for immediate breast reconstruction when it may not be possible for your surgeon to predict whether radiotherapy is going to be required. It's also suitable for women who have large, advanced cancers, when radiotherapy is planned from the outset. Radiotherapy after autologous LD reconstruction occasionally leads to some shrinkage of your reconstructed breast. This shrinkage is most obvious in the upper area of your breast (the cleavage area), but can be corrected by fat transfer.

Disadvantages of the autologous LD flap reconstruction

Disadvantages of the autologous LD flap include a 'donor scar' on your back, which can sometimes be avoided by use of keyhole techniques. There may be a difference between the colour of the skin island (taken from your back) and the remaining skin of your breast. When this 'patch effect' happens, your reconstructed breast will have a patch of paler skin in the centre, surrounded by a rim of darker skin. There may also be a limit to the amount of skin and soft tissue that can be transferred, so that your reconstructed breast may be quite a lot smaller than your other side.

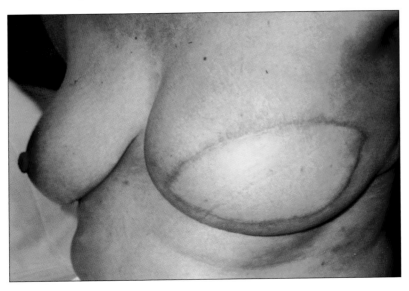

'Patch effect' of the LD skin island

Scars on your back following autologous LD flaps are sometimes slow to heal, and the quality of the scar cannot always be predicted. Even so, these problems compare favourably with some of the abdominal problems experienced by patients after reconstruction with pedicled or free TRAM flaps (see p. 73).

> ❝ I work in a male environment and the guys on the shop floor were a bit dubious about me going to see them afterwards. I don't know whether they thought that I was going to be physically different. As soon as I went in, they all wanted to know what had happened as long as I was happy to tell them. I think that it helped them and me to talk.
>
> My back was a little bit numb where the muscle was moved and even after a year, I have not got full sensitivity, particularly in the front. It used to upset me but does not worry me now. I also used to be able to touch the muscle in my breast and feel the sensation in my back where the muscle had been. I was warned about this but it is strange. It is going away now. ❞

" I had my first mastectomy in 1985 and the second in 1999. I would not have even thought about breast reconstruction if the breast care nurse had not talked to me about it after the second mastectomy. I looked at the leaflets and thought I couldn't possibly think about it at that stage. After I had worn two prostheses for some time and found them pretty awful, I got the leaflets about reconstruction out again. It didn't even dawn on me that I might not consider reconstruction at 62.

I talked to my family doctor and came to the conclusion that I would have reconstruction done using the muscles from my back. My husband took part in the discussions and said that if I wanted reconstruction, I should go ahead. It was an easy decision to make.

I was advised to bring two good quality sports bras and back extensions into hospital with me. It was a wonderful operation and I was not aware of having pain at all. I was out of bed the next day and sat on a seat for a shower after two days. I looked after myself, with all the drains after three days on the ward and it was all manageable. My back was pretty numb, so lying down was no problem. My back is still numb now, three years later but I realise that is just part of the operation. People should be advised to rub cream into the back scars daily because I didn't and it stiffened up a bit. Regular gentle exercises relieve the stiffness.

I went home after a week and could do most things apart from anything heavy. I did the exercises I had been taught regularly.

Once the drains had been removed, I did have fluid collecting on my back, where the muscles had been moved. This is normal and I had it drawn off regularly. This went on for some time. I drove after about three weeks.

It is three years since the reconstructions and there is nothing that I can't do. I can even do curling. In curling, you use your right hand but you have to brush with both hands and it is good exercise to do the sweeping. Nothing is impossible.

I had assumed that having both breasts done, they would both be exactly the same. What I didn't take into account was that the mastectomy scars were different ages and the skin coming in would be at different levels. They did their best with me but it was like working with two different things. I would say that expectations go with age. Even if you have a delayed reconstruction like I did and have a seam, it still looks good wearing a low neckline.

People should take each day as it comes because there will come a day when they forget that they had anything done. I preferred to know as little as possible. It was only the night before the operation when I wondered why I was putting myself through it. I considered going home but thought that everyone would think I was a coward if I walked out. I am glad that I decided to stay and have it done. I have never looked back.

99

Comparing autologous and implant-based LD flap reconstruction at a glance		
	Autologous LD flap	*Implant-based LD flap*
Advantages	All your own tissue	Less surgery on back
	Avoids implants or expanders	Smaller scars on back
	'Ages' very well	Better healing of back
	Tolerates radiotherapy	Adjustable breast size
	Feels warm and lifelike	Good breast shape
	Good for small or medium sized breasts	Suitable for any breast size
Disadvantages	Can shrink	Implant-associated problems: infection, implant loss, 'capsule' formation, implant rupture
	May need modelling by 'lipomodelling'	
	Larger back scar	Need for subsequent implant surveillance and exchange
	Greater risk with back wound problems	
	More fluid collection and 'fat necrosis'	Adverse effects of radiotherapy in up to 50% of women
	Insufficient tissue for more than 30% of women	

5

Reconstruction with a transverse rectus abdominus myocutaneous (TRAM) flap

- **TRAM flap reconstruction uses tissue from your tummy.**
- **You need to be healthy, with a big enough tummy to reconstruct your breast.**
- **You will have the most natural feeling breast reconstruction of all.**
- **It involves major, technically demanding surgery which can weaken your tummy wall.**
- **A free flap has less effect on your tummy wall than a pedicled flap.**
- **Recovery takes about eight to twelve weeks.**
- **Other free flaps can be used in very slim patients who don't have enough tummy tissue to reconstruct their breast.**

The transverse rectus abdominus myocutaneous (TRAM) flap is taken from the lower part of the abdominal wall. It may be 'pedicled' or 'free', and because it removes excess tissue from the lower part of the abdomen, it produces a 'tummy tuck' effect.

Pedicled TRAM flap reconstruction

The pedicled TRAM flap moves the lower abdominal tissue into the breast area, still attached to the blood vessels coming from under the ribs which are channelled along a strip of abdominal muscle – the rectus abdominus or 'rectus' muscle – into the flap. The TRAM flap can produce a breast that has a very natural weight, feel and movement. But it's a complicated and specialised operation that can take your surgical team anything from three to six hours to complete. Because of this, it should only be undertaken by surgeons who are fully trained and skilled in the technique.

The TRAM flap is a major undertaking both for you and your surgeon, but it can result in a very lifelike breast with a natural softness, warmth and feel. If you decide to have your nipple reconstructed later, this is a 'finishing touch' that often makes your breast look and feel even more natural. Many women find that the loss of their tummy is a bonus. The long scar is seen as an acceptable trade-off for a much flatter abdominal wall. You'll also find that your reconstructed breast will gain or lose weight in step with the rest of your body. A natural droop or 'ptosis' of your reconstruction will develop as time goes by. This helps to match your natural breast without having to undertake any further surgery to keep you looking balanced.

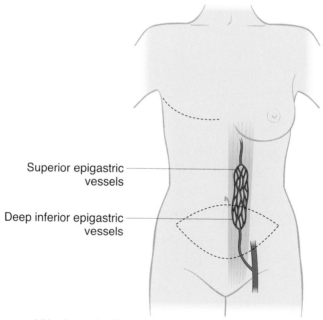

Superior epigastric vessels

Deep inferior epigastric vessels

Anatomy and blood supply of a rectus muscle of the abdominal wall

Deciding if pedicled TRAM flap reconstruction is one of your options

Whether or not a TRAM flap is the right operation for you is a matter for discussion between you and your surgeon. You'll need to have enough fatty tissue on the lower part of your tummy wall to match the size of the breast that's going to be rebuilt. A woman with a slim abdomen isn't suitable for a TRAM flap, because there isn't enough tissue, and there's no point in carrying out this kind of major surgery only to have to use an implant as well. Some women have enough fatty tissue to be able to reconstruct both breasts, and this approach can be very useful if you're facing bilateral mastectomy, maybe to reduce your risk of breast cancer. But your surgeon will have to be sure that you have enough tissue, and that you're fit enough to withstand this type of surgery.

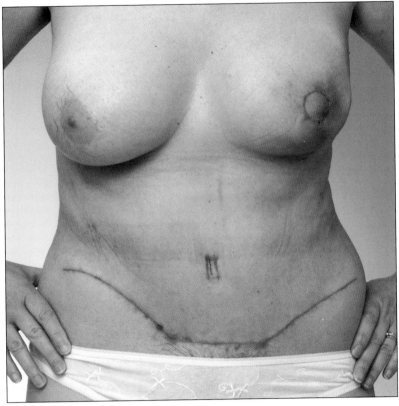

Immediate reconstruction of the left breast with a TRAM flap

The surgery is highly complex and specialised. The blood supply to the flap can be precarious, so a TRAM flap isn't normally recommended for women who are otherwise in poor health. If you're markedly overweight, suffer from high blood pressure or diabetes, or have certain types of abdominal scars, or smoke, then doing a TRAM flap may be too risky and another approach should be considered. If you're a smoker, the arteries that supply your tissues can be narrowed and hardened, and this may result in your flap dying off soon after your operation because of a poor blood supply. So you can see that a TRAM flap isn't a sensible choice for quite a lot of women.

> I was given the choice of three different types of reconstruction – one with an implant, one with the muscle from my back and a TRAM flap. I chose the TRAM flap because I did not want to have an implant.

> The fact that I could have reconstruction done at the same time as the mastectomy was a bonus because I did not want to have any time when I was not complete.
>
> I thought hard about the TRAM flap because it is a more complex operation with a longer recovery period. There are also more things that can go wrong. The latissimus dorsi operation would have involved an implant and when he said that they replace them every ten years, I thought 'That's it. I'm not going through that again. If I have the TRAM flap, it is all my own body.' Although I was going to lose stomach muscle, which is needed, I decided to make that choice. My work as a librarian wasn't a consideration because I have a supportive employer and colleagues.
>
> I did speak to another lady who had a TRAM flap and she was very helpful. She told me that she had no regrets. She was very fit and runs marathons and skis. She said that she would do it again. She told me what to take into hospital, what I would be able to do afterwards and that I should be aware of just how much energy I would lose after the operation. You have to accept that it will be some time before you are anything like back to normal. At least if you are not feeling too well, you know that is to be expected.

> I opted to have a lumpectomy first for breast cancer and was devastated after that when I was told that I needed a mastectomy. I couldn't entertain the idea of a breast reconstruction at that stage, although it was mentioned. I started

to think about the options for reconstruction once the chemotherapy was out of the way. I didn't like myself at all after the mastectomy and found the prosthesis heavy. I made myself go swimming but didn't feel happy.

I didn't know a lot about breast reconstruction but read the information I was given and found it really helpful talking to another person who had reconstruction. I would recommend that to others. I had the choice of reconstruction using a muscle from my back and an implant, or a TRAM flap. I was adamant that if I had reconstruction, I didn't want anything foreign put back into me. I had a lot of discussion with the surgeon and the Breast Care Nurse and was told that the TRAM flap was the most serious operation that I could go for. I was told that the scar on my abdomen would go from hip to hip but it would be quite low down. It took at least twelve months to accept that I was going to have a reconstruction. I chose the TRAM flap.

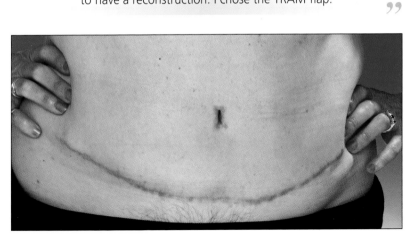

Abdominal scar after a TRAM flap operation

Surgical techniques

The TRAM flap can be used to reconstruct your breast either at the same time as your mastectomy (immediate reconstruction) or at a later date (delayed reconstruction). Not all women are suitable for immediate breast reconstruction, but when it can be done, the overall shape of your reconstructed breast and its sensation is often better than after delayed reconstruction. After a TRAM flap, there's a large scar in the lower part of your tummy, shaped rather like a 'smile', which stretches from hip to hip below your tummy button. The lower the scar, the better the cosmetic result. There will also be a scar around your tummy button, as it needs to be moved into a new position during your surgery.

You'll need to stay in hospital afterwards for anything between four and eight days, depending on your recovery rate and any complications. It's important to stay in hospital while the blood supply to your flap is fully established and until the first stages of healing have taken place. It may be possible to close the gap in your abdominal wall by pulling together the remaining muscles, or by bridging the gap where your rectus muscle has been removed using a sheet of artificial mesh. The rectus muscle is one of several muscles that you use for sitting up – it forms a major part of the 'pedicle' because it helps to carry the blood vessels to the flap, in the flap's 'umbilical cord' (see p. 79).

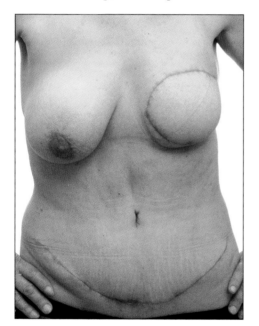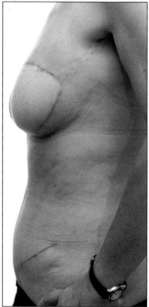

Delayed reconstruction of the left breast using a TRAM flap

A TRAM flap can also be carried out as a delayed reconstruction, many months after your mastectomy. Any poor quality skin from a previous mastectomy scar, or following radiotherapy, can be removed and replaced with healthy skin from your abdomen as part of the

TRAM procedure. When you're having one breast reconstructed, the TRAM flap can be developed either from the same side as the mastectomy, or from the other side. This is called a 'unipedicled' TRAM flap, as it involves one of your two rectus muscles. When it's developed from the same side, there may be a small bulge underneath your breast where the rectus muscle is coming in to supply and nourish the flap. When it's developed on the other side, the bulge may be across the midline in the lower part of your chest, between your breasts. This bulge often shrinks within the first three to six months after surgery, and it's not usually very obvious.

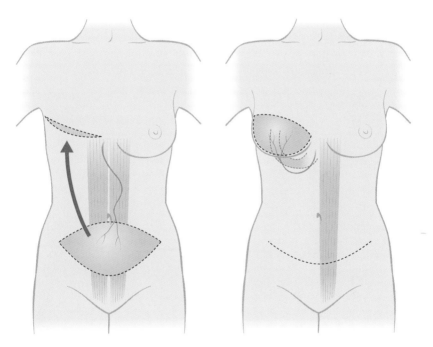

Transposition of a TRAM flap

The scale of your operation and recovery

Initially, your tummy will be tight, and your bed will be flexed at your hips to make you feel more comfortable. Drains will be used for the abdominal wound and also for the breast site. Your room will be kept warm and you'll find it difficult to stand straight in the early days after surgery. You'll begin to mobilise early on, and you may well experience abdominal tightness, which will ease with time.

You're likely to have a small catheter in your bladder to help you pass urine without having to get up to use the toilet. The catheter also allows very careful monitoring of your body fluids and kidney function, both of which are important for good recovery. Your surgeon may advise you to wear leg stockings or to have injections to thin your blood. This is because your surgery takes a long time, and you're likely to spend the early days in bed. During the early stages of your recovery, pain will be kept to a minimum using a number of techniques, including patient-controlled analgesia (PCA). It's important that any pain is kept at bay to build up your confidence and to get you going as soon as possible after your surgery.

If you're having both breasts reconstructed, then your surgeon may decide to use both rectus muscles, a so-called 'bipedicled' TRAM flap. When your flap is harvested, it's left attached to both muscles and then divided in half. So each half is supplied with blood from its own pedicle or 'umbilical' cord, and is used to reconstruct one of the missing breasts.

A TRAM flap is a long operation, and there will be some blood loss. This will make you feel tired for some weeks after surgery while you restore your own levels. Blood transfusion is rarely required. If you're undergoing any major surgery such as reconstruction of both of your breasts, it may be possible for you to donate some of your blood a few weeks in advance. This can then be stored and given back to you during your operation – an 'auto-transfusion'.

> 66 I found it hard to move when I first woke up after the operation. There were drains, a drip and it felt sore rather than painful. I sat in the chair after three days and had to use every single muscle in my body just to stay upright. When I first started walking, I felt as though I had lead weights on the end of my legs. I found it shocking looking at the breast and tummy scar at first but now I don't take any notice of it at all. The exercises were painful but it became easier. Doing a little bit at a time helps you to get a bit further.
>
> The most difficult things to do at first were walking because the scar went from hip to hip and reaching for things. I couldn't do an awful lot for the first month. I managed to walk around the house and up and down the stairs. Now and again I tried something more difficult. After that, I started looking after the

house. I felt like a fraud and didn't like accepting help because I was used to doing a busy cleaning job as well as doing everything for my family. Once the pulling sensation went, it was much easier. It took a good six months to get back to my usual activities but I did have chemotherapy in that time.

Sometimes, I just did not want the family to see me and I just didn't feel like myself but I got over it in time. They were just feelings that you go through. I do go dancing again now and love that. Having my family around me helped me get through it and they need me now just as much as before, even my new grandchild does.

99

66

Because of the long anaesthetic, I wasn't too with it for the rest of the day after the operation. All the things like oxygen, drainage bottles and a drip were manageable. It was four days before I got to the bathroom on my own. When you take your first steps, you feel the stitches pulling in your abdomen. It wasn't painful, just very uncomfortable.

I looked at my new breast as soon as I was conscious enough. I was impressed with it and it was a relief to see it. My husband was also impressed when I showed him in hospital.

I blow-dried my hair with the affected arm and I could get washed and walk across the ward to talk to people after five days. I went home after a week.

I couldn't do a lot when I first went home. My husband did the cooking and looked after me. One of the main things that strikes you is how tired you get. You very quickly find out that you can't do what you thought you could. It is easy to become impatient. I found that I got used to it and settled into making the most of being at home.

I drove again after two months. That wasn't purely because of the physical side. I felt that because I had been out of it for so long, I wasn't sure that I was up to speed mentally.

I went back to work after ten months and had a staggered return. I have been back at work full-time for a year and I do get tired sometimes but I think that I would have done anyway. I have quite a demanding job. There are no practical things that I still find difficult.

The reconstruction has given me a very natural appearance. I am confident in my dress and day-to-day life. If I had to, I would do the same again.

" I had to stay in bed for the first three days after the reconstruction and the worst thing was that they had to keep me really warm. I suffered from hot flushes because the chemotherapy had put me through an early menopause. I had no problems with my breast and didn't have a lot of feeling in it. My tummy was the worst part to get over. It was painful for the first three weeks but improved after that. My first walk in hospital was awful because it was very painful but once I had done that, things got better.

It was hard initially at home. Walking up the stairs was difficult but the more I did it, the easier it became. My husband was at home to help me. I started to do more around the house after six weeks and the wound healed up really well. I did no heavy lifting for some time. I found that swimming was very helpful.

The breasts match pretty well and are excellent in a bra. The reconstructed breast is not quite as full as the other in one place and I am careful about some tops I wear. Everybody tells me that you can't see it from the front. We did discuss having the other breast reduced, depending on how the new breast turned out but this has not been necessary. As far as my tummy is concerned, I have a flat tummy now and that is great. I can wear whatever clothes I like.

My husband has been very supportive and the mastectomy made no difference to him, although it did to me. Even now that I have had the reconstruction, it still makes a bit of difference to me because although I have the shape, there is very little feeling in the breast.

It is now eighteen months since the reconstruction and I can still not stretch up too far. It feels as though there is a weakness in my tummy and my lower back feels as though it has not got the muscle support that it had before. These are not difficulties compared to the psychological benefits of the reconstruction. "

Complications following your surgery

Even with the highest standards of care and attention to detail, complications can and do sometimes occur. Difficulties may be encountered while the new tissues are healing into place. Very occasionally, the flap will fail totally, but this happens in fewer than 4% of women. Even so, it's important that you realise it's a rare possibility. Sometimes the blood supply to the flap may be just enough to keep it alive, but not good enough to keep the tissue soft and healthy. When this happens, hardness may develop in the fatty tissue, known as 'fat necrosis'. This may feel quite like a tumour, but your surgeon will be able to reassure you and it will usually settle and soften with time. Liposuction can also help to treat it.

If bleeding continues after your operation into the spaces over your tummy or around your new breast, a 'haematoma' or collection of blood can develop. This usually settles by itself, but occasionally your surgeon will need to take you back to theatre to stop the bleeding and to clear away the haematoma. In the long term, your abdomen may be weakened by the operation, and an abdominal hernia can occasionally result. In a significant proportion of women, full sensation in the lower part of the tummy may never recover. Because of this, you should be particularly careful to avoid undue heat to the skin of the lower part of your abdomen, such as a hot-water bottle or lying in very hot sun.

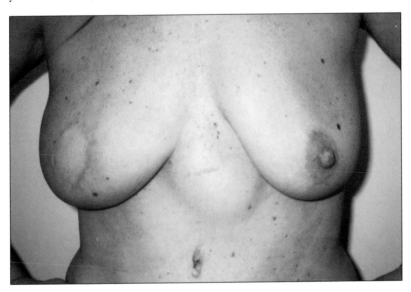

Abdominal hernia after a pedicled TRAM flap reconstruction

" During the first year, I began to feel as though there was a knot in my tummy sometimes. I mentioned it and was told at first that it would improve. I also had some bulging of the scar on the side where most of the operation had been. It got worse and worse and I went back to see the surgeon who told me he thought that I had a hernia and it would need repairing. In a strange way, I was relieved to be told that it was a complication of the surgery because it had been getting so uncomfortable and it was nice to know that something could be done to get rid of it.

I had the hernia repair 18 months after the breast reconstruction. It involved opening up my tummy scar again and they also moved my tummy button. It was not quite as big an operation as the reconstruction and my recovery was remarkably good. I was in hospital for a week. I could move about at home but I was a bit doubled up as before because of the pulling stitches. It wasn't too bad. I just had to be careful about lifting again. I had about a month off work. When I went back, I could do everything apart from picking up huge boxes of brochures from the floor.

It took two years to fully recover from the reconstruction and the hernia repair. Nearly three years have passed since the reconstruction and I feel really good. I do feel that it has been worth having the reconstruction, despite the hernia. When the hernia got bad, I wondered why I had bothered with the reconstruction but now I would say that it was definitely the right way to go. "

Recovery from the TRAM flap operation is slower than after other kinds of breast reconstruction. Most women find that they can stand upright by ten to twelve days, and can gradually get back to normal activities after three to four weeks. But you'll find it's difficult to return to full time work in under twelve weeks. You should be able to do gentle sports once your breast and tummy have healed soundly. Your physiotherapist will give you good advice about the exercises you can do to build up your strength and confidence as soon as you've had your operation (see p. 169).

Free TRAM flap reconstruction (DIEP Flap)

Deciding if free TRAM flap reconstruction is one of your options

The 'spare tyre' on the lower abdomen can often provide ample material to reconstruct a new breast without the need for a breast implant. The deep inferior epigastric artery perforator (DIEP) flap allows the reconstruction of one or two larger and more pendulous breasts in women who don't have enough tissue for LD flaps or who need to have a large amount of breast skin replaced. Closure of the gap left in the wall of the abdomen is like having a 'tummy tuck'. This is because it tightens the tissues lying over the lower part of your tummy, leaving a transverse scar from one hip to the other and a small scar around your tummy button (umbilicus).

This type of abdominal tissue breast reconstruction is best for young and active women who want to maintain their sporting lifestyle, women who are planning to have children in the future and those women who require bilateral breast reconstruction. This is because it's able to preserve the strength and function of the abdominal wall as the blood supply is divided completely. But it's only suitable for fit and healthy patients without any additional health problems, because it's a very complex procedure with prolonged recovery time.

Surgical technique

The skin and fat between your tummy button and your groin receives its circulation through blood vessels that originate from the groin. They are called the deep inferior epigastric vessels and travel under and through the two long strap muscles in your abdominal wall (the rectus abdominus or 'rectus' muscles). Smaller branches of these vessels (perforators) then nourish the overlying skin. A second, smaller set of blood vessels (superior epigastric vessels) travel under your breast bone through your chest and connect to the lower deep inferior epigastric vessels within your rectus muscle. This fatty tissue is also nourished by the third set of blood vessels (superficial epigastric vessels), which come from the blood vessels in your thigh, but these may have been damaged by previous surgery in this area, such as hernia repair, varicose vein surgery or caesarean section (see p. 74 for an illustration of blood supply).

The first part of this section described how the pedicled TRAM flap uses the skin and fatty tissue from your lower tummy attached to one or two of your rectus muscles. The pedicled flap is nourished through the superior epigastric vessels which come from your chest, but this weakens your tummy. This can sometimes interfere with lifting, housework, sports and even simple activities such as getting out of bed. Because the rectus muscles counterbalance your back muscles, back problems may also occur after the pedicled TRAM flap. It's also been pointed out that muscle harvest can weaken your abdominal wall with bulging or even hernia formation. The vast majority of these problems can be avoided with the DIEP flap.

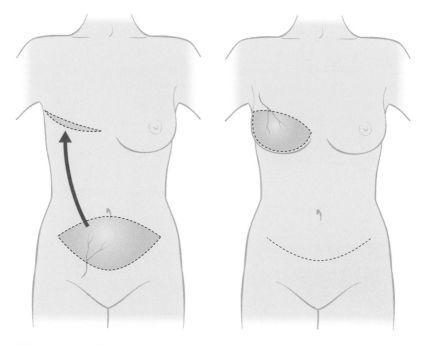

Transposition of the DIEP flap

This type of reconstruction is called a 'free tissue transfer'. Unlike the pedicled TRAM flap, all of the skin and fatty tissue on your lower tummy is disconnected completely and then reconnected to blood vessels in your mastectomy area. This clever technique allows your surgeon to take only what's needed to make your new breast: skin, fat and blood vessels to keep the tissue alive. The small perforating blood vessels are traced through a split in your rectus muscle down to the larger blood vessels – the deep inferior epigastric vessels – in your groin. So the muscles and the strength of your abdominal wall are preserved more or less completely. The blood supply is then disconnected and your flap is then transferred to your chest where your breast is reconstructed. The blood supply to your new breast is re-established by connection of the small blood vessels which have been divided to blood vessels in your axilla (your armpit) or behind your breastbone. This is a very delicate procedure and the join-up has to be done using a microscope as the blood vessels are so small.

The scale of the operation and recovery

Free tissue transfer is a complicated and technically demanding procedure. The perforating blood vessels that are traced through your muscle are only one to two millimetres in diameter and great care has to be taken during the operation to avoid damage to these delicate structures. Equally great care has to be taken during the re-connection of your blood vessels under the microscope. This operation takes approximately six to eight hours to complete and patients will spend one to two weeks in hospital. Most women take two to three months to recover from the operation, before the strength of their tummy muscles has recovered completely.

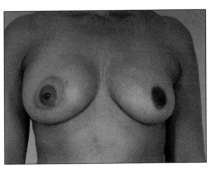 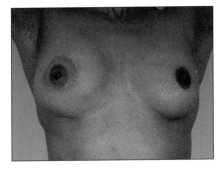

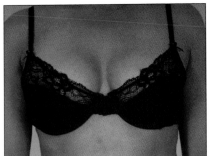 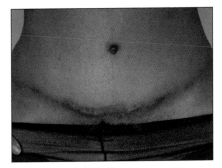

Immediate reconstruction of the right breast with a DIEP flap

The free DIEP flap is a much more involved procedure than the autologous LD flap. It may be a woman's only option for breast reconstruction if there isn't enough tissue on her back or if her LD muscle can't be used because of previous surgery. Other women who are suitable for this type of breast reconstruction are those who need to have a large amount of breast skin removed and replaced because of a large breast cancer, or those who have developed a recurrence of breast cancer after previous lumpectomy and radiotherapy. The free DIEP flap is also suitable for delayed reconstruction of a larger and droopier breast and for women requesting bilateral breast reconstruction because of a high risk of familial breast cancer.

This technique isn't suitable for patients who have significant health problems such as diabetes, heart or lung disease or autoimmune diseases, all of which can interfere with the blood supply to the flap, causing it to die off. Previous operations can also damage these blood vessels as well as the new blood supply in the chest.

Complications following your surgery

Naturally, such a complex procedure involving microsurgery has a higher failure rate than the LD flap or the pedicled TRAM flap, both of which leave the flap tissues connected to their original circulation. The blood vessels of a free flap can clog up, twist or kink and this interferes with the circulation of blood into or out of the flap. This happens in up to one in ten cases. These patients have to go back to theatre immediately so that the surgeon can try to re-establish the circulation to the new breast. This is successful in most cases but if not, then part of the flap or the whole flap may be lost. The overall success rate of the free DIEP flap is about 98% when the surgeon performs this procedure regularly.

Other complications affect the flap itself or the flap donor site. The most common problems are haematoma formation (blood clot in the wound), delayed wound healing, wound infection and fat necrosis (when some of the fatty tissue dies off). Asymmetry of the donor site on the tummy wall is also possible and may need minor revision later on, but bulging and hernia formation are rarer than for women after pedicled TRAM reconstruction.

The need for symmetry surgery and the effects of radiotherapy

It's not always possible to predict the final size and shape of your reconstructed breast and further surgery to your reconstructed breast or the opposite breast may be desired to achieve symmetry. From then on, there's rarely any need for further surgery because breasts made entirely of living tissue behave and react to changes in body weight and gravity just like a natural breast.

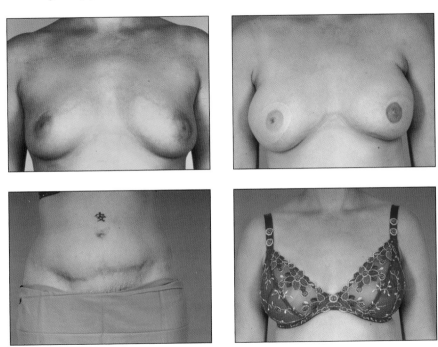

Bilateral reconstruction with DIEP flaps after radiotherapy

On the other hand, the reaction of a breast reconstructed with abdominal tissue to radiotherapy is somewhat unpredictable. All tissues react to radiotherapy just like a real breast does after lumpectomy. Some women show hardly any signs, but others develop a quite marked hardening and shrinkage of their breast. Women with larger, more fatty breasts are more likely to develop a bigger reaction and in the same way, women with large breasts who've had a reconstruction with quite a lot of fatty tissue from the abdomen may also be at higher risk of hardening and shrinkage following treatment. Radiotherapy will also make it impossible for the breast to increase and decrease in size with changes in body weight, and to develop a natural droop over time. Because of these side effects of radiotherapy, it's more than likely that a difference in size and shape of the reconstructed breast will develop over time, so more of these patients need to have symmetry surgery to the other breast as time goes by.

It isn't possible to predict how an individual patient is going to react to radiotherapy. Because of this, some surgeons won't agree to perform this type of surgery at the same time as mastectomy, when the need for radiotherapy can't be judged with certainty, so they may recommend that the reconstruction is delayed until all treatment is finished. What's interesting is that most women are equally happy with their reconstruction in the long term, whether they've had radiotherapy or not. So it's very important to discuss these issues thoroughly with your surgeon before surgery.

> " The second surgeon who I saw agreed with me that because of my large droopy breasts, the DIEP flap would give me a more realistic reconstruction. He said that if I did want to have that, he would refer me to a plastic surgeon who specialised in this. By the time that I saw the plastic surgeon, my mind was made up about the DIEP flap. I realised that mastectomy alone was not for me and I wanted to feel that I was back to being as normal as I could be.
>
> I didn't like the idea of having tissue tunnelled up through my flesh because that makes the muscles not quite as good as they were. I really liked the idea of having the blood supply disconnected and reconnected so that I was left as normal as possible. I didn't like the idea of implants, however safe anybody tells me they are. Somebody else might be quite happy with that.
>
> I was 66 when I had the DIEP flap. When I came round, they said that I was chirpier than people usually are. However, I did feel very knocked out. I was monitored every hour for several days. I remember thinking that I didn't want anyone to do anything to me again. I didn't even want a nipple!
>
> I got up after three days. I was quite constrained by the drips and drains but could do most things with my arm on the reconstructed side. Because the nurses had to keep the reconstructed breast warm, they would check it regularly. That was when I looked at the breast. What I hadn't realised, although

it is quite logical, was that I kept my own skin on the breast. It made me feel as if I had not lost anything.

I went home after nine days. I live on my own and looked after myself. Before going into hospital, I made lots of pre-prepared meals so that I just had to take something out of the freezer and cook a few vegetables to get a meal. You just have to recognise that you do things slowly. I didn't want to be looked after. I had a sleep every day after lunch and a friend shopped for me. I wasn't as fit as I usually am before the operation because it was only about two months after I had finished chemotherapy and that was very depleting. I think that I would have found it more difficult to cope if I had never had an operation before.

My tummy wound took about four weeks to heal because I had a collection of fluid under the scar which needed to be removed. Although the scar is a very long one, I could wear a bikini now. My tummy button has been moved sideways slightly and although I would prefer it to be in the middle, it doesn't seem to be a big issue.

I restarted driving after nearly five weeks. Although my tummy felt numb to touch, when I went over bumps in the road, it felt incredibly sensitive. My arm was not a problem.

I had two and a half months off work. I was held up by the slow healing of my tummy scar. By the time that I was back at work, I was doing normal things around the house. I do still get tired and hope this will improve.

I go to the gym and do as much of my exercise programme as I feel able at the time.

I have had to have another small operation to take a tuck in the reconstructed breast to make the shape match better. I may need to have this done again. I don't mind about having these procedures done because it only involves having a local anaesthetic.

It is now seven months since the reconstruction and my new breast doesn't droop quite as much as the other one. I have got used to that and it is near enough the same. I would not want to have any adjustments made to the other breast. It doesn't look any different in a bra because I use a silk scarf to pad the bra out. I knew that I would be pleased that I had the reconstruction, even immediately after the operation. I made a clear decision about what kind of operation I wanted. It was the right thing for me to do. ""

" I found it very hard after the operation because I was in a room on my own and had to lie flat on my back. I am not a person who likes to sit still. There were lots of drips and drains and I controlled the painkillers, which was all right. You have to be very careful with the affected arm in case you damage the blood vessels. I got out of bed after three or four days and because the arm was weak, it was helpful to have things where I could reach them. I went home after two weeks.

I found it very difficult to do much at home. This was partly because of the tummy scar which ran from side to side. I had already had two caesarean sections, so it meant just making the scar bigger. I found walking hard and getting to the shops at the top of the road after two weeks at home was an achievement. I always had someone with me who could carry the shopping. If I had little goals, it made me do a bit more each time.

I went back to work after six months part-time to begin with and gradually built it up until I did a full day's work. You want to get back to a normal routine and in reality there is no way that you can do this straightaway. It is tiring and I was frightened that people would knock me. We were asked to wear a sports bra from the first day, to support the reconstructed breast and I have found it more comfortable to continue doing that since.

Initially, the reconstructed breast was much bigger than the other one, partly due to the swelling. After that settled, it was still larger than the other breast. The surgeon told me that the size of the reconstructed breast could be reduced when I had the nipple reconstruction. It is a good idea to talk to the surgeon about the expected size of the breast before the operation. ""

" I was given a choice of three different breast reconstructions which I could have at the same time as the mastectomy. My partner was involved from day one and that was very helpful for both of us. I liked the idea of having something that was made from me and was as natural as it could be, so I chose to have the DIEP flap.

For the first couple of days after the reconstruction I felt as though I had been hit by several buses. I also felt relieved and exhausted. I was mentally exhausted because there is a big run up to something major like that. I watched the other girls who had the same operation as me and they looked as wrecked as I did for the first couple of days. I was moving into my chair by the third day and the big milestone was having the urinary catheter taken out and going to the bathroom. The physiotherapy helped with my arm movements and I was able to stretch my arm out properly after some time.

I developed an MRSA infection in my wound and that delayed my recovery. I had to go back into hospital for treatment twice and that was distressing. If it hadn't been for that, the whole procedure would have been so smooth and I would have been back at work quite quickly.

I have a numb sensation under my arm on the side that was reconstructed. I am getting used to it: it feels odd putting on deodorant and sometimes you scratch your arm in one place and get a funny sensation in another part of the arm. It feels odd but not horrible.

I wish that I had had the tummy scar put in a different place. When I spoke to the surgeon before the operation, she told me to wear a pair of knickers that I like to wear and then we could work out how high or low to put the scar. I didn't listen to her properly and wore the wrong pair and wish that I had thought more about it. I could have had the scar a bit lower. It is totally up to you and you know what you like to wear. After she had done all the drawings on me, I wondered whether I could say anything and I wish now that I had. It makes no odds to the surgeons and they want you to be happy with the result of the surgery. It would have been a simple thing to do.

My whole shape has changed since having a DIEP flap made. I used to have a small waist and big hips. Now, my waist size has gone up a bit but I have a flat tummy, which I like.

My partner is fine with the reconstruction. It doesn't bother him at all. He is not worried about touching or caressing it the way he does with the other one. At first, he was worried about touching me in general, in case it was a bit sore but now, it is no problem. I feel great about the future now and am glad that the breast problem was caught early. I feel that I am healthier now than I was in the first place.
"

"
I was told that a DIEP flap tends to give a more realistic looking breast. When you are dealing with body fat as opposed to an implant, you have more leeway to mould it and make it look more natural. That was a priority for me. I decided to go for the more natural look and have the DIEP flap, although it was a bigger operation.

I was fine immediately after the operation. There was no pain in the breast region, it was totally numb. The pain in my abdominal scar was just like a really bad period pain. I could have had morphine for pain control but I did not have any. I felt fine emotionally.

I think that I had to stay in bed for five days. I had to keep still for the first two days, which was hard. The blanket to keep the breast reconstruction warm was uncomfortably hot. The heat made me itchy and it is helpful to use some baby powder. It is a good idea to put long hair up before the operation because you get hot lying for so long. I used a V-shaped pillow under my arms and one under my legs to stop the tummy scar pulling when I was resting.

By the time that I went home after a week, I was feeding myself with the other hand. I started walking about after four days and it felt quite strange. I tended to want to shuffle, as opposed to walking properly. The surgeon was very strict about how much I should do with the arm on the reconstructed side, in case I damaged the blood vessels which had been joined under my arm.

I think that I could do most things at home. I made sure that I could put my make-up on with my left hand. I started to use the arm more after the first week. My husband has always been the homemaker but nobody did any more for me than they would normally have done. I was determined to get up and about. Because I wore an abdomen binder for some time after the operation, I was unable to fit into normal skirts. Elasticated waistbands are helpful. I drove after four weeks because I was keen to do so. My family were amazed.

I had chemotherapy after the operation and it is now a year since the reconstruction. I started going to the gym a few months ago and I do rowing and things like that. Exercise doesn't feel any different than it did before. The arm on the reconstructed side feels as strong as the other one.

I have a totally flat stomach below the navel and a thin white line where my briefs go. I wore a bikini in the summer and haven't done that for years.

The reconstruction itself looks brilliant and that is a combination of the surgeon's skill and the fact that I kept my own skin and nipple. I am really proud of it and don't think that I shall ever take my body for granted. I don't feel any less confident than I was before. If anything, more so.

"

" Ten months after having a DIEP flap, the reconstruction started to go wrong. It appears to have sunk inwards on the lower part and felt hard, although the cleavage was still fine. I was told that I had fat necrosis and needed to have the lower part of the breast refashioned. To begin with, it didn't bother me and I was in two minds about whether to have this done because I had gone back to work, been promoted and it felt like a step backwards. The plastic surgeon said that because I was young and have all those years ahead of me, I wouldn't be happy later if it was not done, and that it might be better to get it done in case it got any worse.

I had a second operation which removed all the hard fat and was supposed to pull up some surplus fat from beneath my reconstructed breast to fill in the area. This was not at all successful and left me with a strange lumpy mound which wouldn't hold a bra in place and was uncomfortable. It was then recommended that I had a further reconstruction with a silicone implant and I decided to go ahead with this.

"

Comparing pedicled and free TRAM flap reconstructions at a glance		
	Pedicled TRAM flap	**Free TRAM flap**
Advantages	All your own tissue	All your own tissue
	Soft, warm, natural breast	Soft, warm, natural breast
	Breast matures with age	Breast matures with age
	Breast mirrors your weight	Breast mirrors your weight
	Gives you a 'tummy tuck'	Gives you a 'tummy tuck'
		Doesn't weaken your abdomen
		Doesn't affect your back
		Avoids hernias
Disadvantages	Health problems prevent	Health problems prevent
	Four to six hours surgery	Six to eight hours surgery
	Specialist skill required	Microvascular skill required
	Blood supply problems in 4%	Blood supply problems in 10%
	Long scar on tummy	Long scar on tummy
	Three months off work	Two to three months off work
	Hernias and 'bulging'	
	Back problems	Variable radiotherapy tolerance
	Variable radiotherapy tolerance	

Alternative types of free flaps

Some very slim women have no spare tissue at all on their backs or abdomen. If they need or request a breast reconstruction with their own tissue, this can be taken from other sites, such as the buttocks, hips and thighs.

The superior gluteal artery perforator flap (SGAP) and inferior gluteal artery perforator flap (IGAP) are free flaps of skin and fat that are taken from the buttocks. Perforating blood vessels are traced through the muscles on your buttocks to the underlying larger blood vessels called the superior and inferior gluteal arteries. These blood vessels are divided and then connected to blood vessels behind your breastbone. The amount of tissue that can be transferred with these techniques is limited, but fortunately most very slim patients also have relatively small breasts. The scar is usually hidden under your pants, and a certain amount of asymmetry of your buttocks is common unless both breasts are reconstructed. Bilateral breast reconstructions may require two separate procedures. Each side involves a six to eight hour operation, one to two weeks in hospital and six to eight weeks' recovery. Most patients do not experience any restrictions in their everyday lives because no muscle is removed during the procedure.

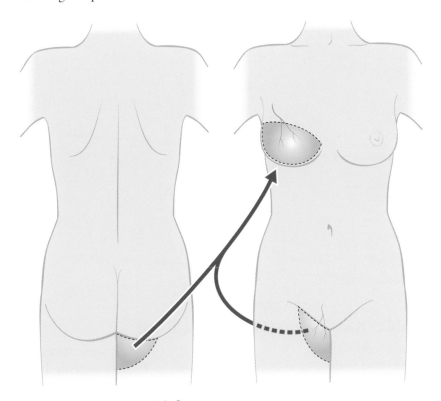

Reconstruction using TUG flap

Other donor sites for free flap breast reconstruction also include the saddlebag area of the thighs (lateral transverse thigh flap: LTT), the inner aspect of the thighs (transverse upper gracilis flap: TUG) and the so-called 'Rubens flap', which uses the 'love handles' over the hips.

Although the buttocks are probably the most popular alternative to the DIEP free flap, there aren't very many surgeons in the UK who regularly perform these operations. So it's wise to be referred to a surgeon with plenty of experience if you're considering one of these procedures. The DIEP flap from the abdomen is routine for most reconstructive micro-surgeons with success rates of about 98%. Free tissue transfer from the buttocks or from the thighs is much less common and the success rates are lower. If you're considering any of these alternatives, it is very important to have a thorough discussion with your surgeons about all specific risks and the success rate of the particular centre.

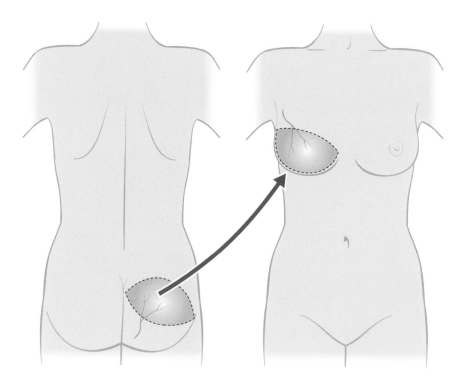

Reconstruction using SGAP flap

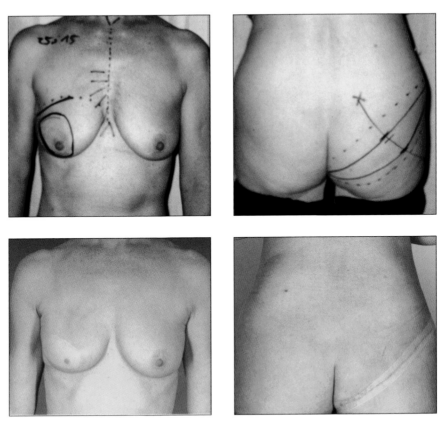

Right breast reconstruction using SGAP flap

> 66 I was just 50 when I was told I needed a mastectomy but could have a breast reconstruction as well. The plastic surgeon said that I didn't have enough fat on my stomach to use that muscle, so the options were: a silicone implant, taking some muscle from my back or taking some of my buttock and using that. I was slim and very conscious of my body and wanted to get the best result if I was going to have a reconstruction done. I lead a really young lifestyle, going clubbing and dancing, and my body image is important to me.

I wasn't keen on silicone because I wanted something more natural. I was told that the most natural result would be from the reconstruction using part of my buttock. The thing against the SGAP reconstruction was that it would take eight hours. I was terrified of an operation that was that long. I was told that the scars from the SGAP would be inside my bikini line and that my buttock wouldn't look that different, partly because I have a small bust and they would not have to take too much tissue. I spoke to someone who was able to reassure me about the long anaesthetic and then decided to have the SGAP reconstruction.

I had to lie flat for the first day after the operation. There were drains to the breast and my buttock. When I got up to the lavatory I had to manage with a drip stand, an arm that I couldn't bend and take off really tight support pants. I was doing that from the second day after the operation.

I went home after five days. Although I couldn't walk far by then, I was keen to get home. A friend looked after me to begin with. I had to wear a heavy-duty bra and support pants for six months, which I hated. The buttock was never much of a problem. It didn't hurt much.

I am fit and supple from doing yoga but found not being able to do things like lift my arm far quite frustrating. Things like shopping on my own were difficult at first. Using a trolley or a suitcase on wheels was helpful. You need to be prepared for several months of recovery and do have to take it easy. It is helpful to have somebody supporting you at home in the first few weeks.

By five weeks after the operation, I went to a concert in the Students' Union with my son which involved standing up all evening and I enjoyed it!

I went back to work part-time after three months and found that I was too tired to do much after work. I work in IT, so once I had got there, I just had to sit there and do the work. There was no problem with using my arm and the computer but I did notice that my arm was weak for some time. I got into the habit of using the other hand, where possible, for anything heavy. I worked full-time after four months and didn't look back.

I think that I was pretty much back to normal by the time that I got together with my 26-year-old partner eight months after the operation. My confidence was helped by having the reconstruction, rather than a mastectomy.

The reconstructed breast is not the same as a real breast and never will be, but the fact that they used my skin helps. I can feel when something is touching the breast but have no more sensation than that.

We have a busy time and I still get pain under my arm after playing frisbee for a long time. Going to a really hectic ceilidh and being swung around by the arm hurts afterwards for a day or two. It also hurts after windsurfing, but is no worse than after doing exercises. I have also managed a backpacking holiday in Brazil.

I have got a big scar running across my buttock but it does fit inside my bikini line. It doesn't really bother me much. The overall appearance of the reconstructed breast is pretty good. To me, it looks slightly lumpy and not like a normal breast. I don't think that the shape has changed in the past two years.

If I had to have breast reconstruction again, I would probably go for the same thing. Life is great. It is not the end of the world and life should go on. You can still enjoy life afterwards. 99

6 Reconstruction after partial mastectomy

- Reconstruction after partial mastectomy is a new and increasingly popular option for patients.

- This procedure isn't suitable for everyone.

- There are two different approaches that can be used depending on the size of your breast.

- A partial reconstruction is a smaller operation than a full reconstruction.

- Your reconstructed breast normally looks and feels like part of you.

Until recently, surgeons treating breast cancer were only able to offer their patients one or two choices – either breast-conserving surgery (lumpectomy) or mastectomy, with or without immediate reconstruction. This is because if your surgeon has to remove much more than a fifth of your breast tissue then the gap left behind is usually very obvious, making the breast look distorted. So a mastectomy is often a better option in this situation. The chances of lumpectomy causing obvious deformity depend not only on the proportion of the breast that has been removed, but also the part of the breast that has been taken away. The most obvious and distressing deformities follow removal of large amounts of tissue from the central, inner and lower parts of the breast. So when a lot of tissue has to be removed the surgeon usually advises mastectomy and an external prosthesis or a full reconstruction. Reconstruction is a good solution, but often requires major surgery.

Development of a new approach

A new approach has been developed recently that offers another choice to women who until now would have been advised to have a mastectomy because of the amount of tissue they would lose. This new approach offers patients the opportunity to have the 'gap' in their breast reconstructed with their own tissue. This is normally done at the same time as the surgery to remove the tumour, so the shape and the appearance of the breast aren't destroyed.

Surgeons doing this innovative type of surgery have to be skilled in techniques for removing the cancer, as well as being familiar with the techniques for reconstructing the 'gap'. This may mean that two surgeons – a breast surgeon and a plastic surgeon – will need to do the operation together, working as a team. But it can be difficult to organise this because surgeons normally have different timetables. Fortunately, more surgeons are becoming multi-skilled, and many Breast Units today are supported by 'oncoplastic' surgeons. These specialists are trained not only to remove the cancer, but also to rebuild the area that has been taken away.

This approach isn't suitable for everyone, but it's becoming an increasingly popular choice as it allows a greater number of women to avoid a full mastectomy. There are some other advantages too. Rebuilding part of the breast involves less extensive surgery than reconstructing the whole breast, and some of the complications of reconstruction with breast implants are avoided, including the adverse effects that radiotherapy can have on the tissues around implants and expanders. Only the diseased part of the breast has been removed – the rest of the breast feels and looks entirely normal – and because there is less surgery, there is a smaller risk of developing complications.

> 66 I am glad that I was able to keep some of the breast. I remember thinking before the operation that this was the last time that I was going to be normal. However, it is still me, my nipple, my breast and back. I am glad that I made that decision. I still would not want to wake up without the breast. 99

Choice of technique

There are two different ways that a surgeon can reconstruct your breast after partial mastectomy (the term used when a large amount of breast tissue is removed).

- **Volume replacement**

  The tissue that has been removed is replaced with tissue borrowed from another part of your body. After this kind of surgery, your reconstructed breast should be very similar in size and shape to your other breast.

- **Volume displacement**

  The tissue from another part of your breast is moved into the gap to fill and reconstruct it. After this kind of surgery, the breast will have a good shape, but it will be smaller than the other side because the tissue that has been removed has not been replaced by tissue from elsewhere. Instead, it has been borrowed from the breast itself. Because of this, very often another operation to reduce the size of the other breast is necessary to achieve a match.

Volume replacement procedures

During volume replacement operations your surgeon will usually borrow tissue from the muscle on your back (your latissimus dorsi (LD) muscle), together with a layer of fatty tissue overlying the muscle. Sometimes a small island of skin will be taken attached to the muscle if it has been necessary to take skin away from the breast. The amount

Volume replacement procedures

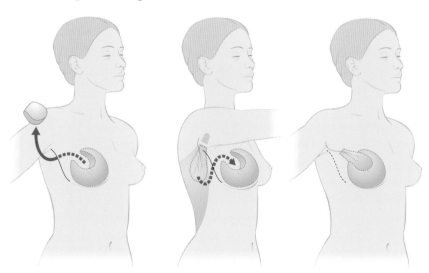

LD miniflap without a skin island

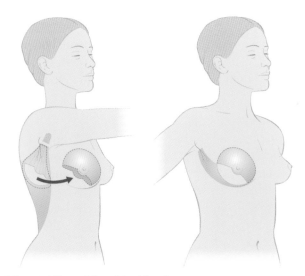

LD miniflap with a skin island

of tissue needed to fill the gap in the breast is usually smaller than the amount of tissue needed to reconstruct the whole breast when a full mastectomy has been carried out. This is why the flap is called a 'miniflap'. This flap is then swung through your armpit and is 'shaped' to fit into the gap in your breast. The muscle is able to contract and small movements can sometimes be seen under the skin where it lies in the breast. Very often your nipple won't have to be removed.

<blockquote>
" The first thing that I remember asking after the operation was whether I still had a nipple. I had. By the time that I went home from hospital, I could do most light things around the house. I was quite into sport at the time of the operation; I was running up until two days beforehand. I therefore didn't feel ill and I felt a bit down because I couldn't go running afterwards. I can remember a friend coming to see me and telling me that I was holding my arm rigidly. It was because of that I realised that I should do more exercises. I then regularly did the exercises I had already been given and it improved.

I just have a scar line running down the side of the breast from the armpit and underneath the breast. Nobody would know that
</blockquote>

it was there unless I was to go around with my arm up in the air. The reconstructed breast is a better shape than the other breast. It is only really noticeable when you are lying flat on your back. My natural breast is firmer than the other. The shape has not really changed over the past five years. I have a slight dent in the top of my breast but I have never worn really low tops. That is manageable.

Scars in patients after LD miniflap operations

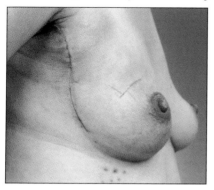
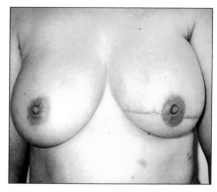

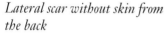

Lateral scar without skin from the back

Breast scar with skin from the back

Occasionally, fatty tissue alone may be borrowed from the armpit when there is enough tissue here to reconstruct the gap. Volume replacement operations are most suitable for women with small or medium-sized breasts who don't want to drop one or two bra sizes as a result of their surgery. If your surgeon doesn't have to take any skin from your back, you'll have a single scar running down the outer side of your breast. If skin is needed for the reconstruction, you'll have a scar on your breast and on one side of your back.

Volume displacement procedures

Women with larger, heavier breasts are more likely to be advised to consider a volume displacement operation. This will reduce the overall size and weight of the breast. Because of this, a 'mirror image' operation removing the same amount of tissue from the other breast will give the patient a smaller, balanced bust. These operations are modelled on a variety of well-established techniques that are normally used for breast reduction operations. Breast reduction is a common procedure for

106

women who are handicapped by the abnormally large size of their breasts. The surgeon can adapt this procedure to include the removal of the cancer in the middle of tissue that is normally taken away to reduce the size of the breast. These skilled approaches can remove the tumour very thoroughly, without causing any distortion. The scars following volume displacement operations run around the nipple and downwards into the fold under the breast. A variety of different techniques can be used, depending on the position and size of the tumour.

> ❝ My scars look like an inverted 'T' shape, running down from each nipple and underneath the breasts from side to side, going slightly up into the armpits. My breasts are a different shape now but not that different. I lost one nipple but I am pleased that I still have one. The surgeon did offer to make another nipple on the right side but I think I was happy with the situation at my age. Maybe if I was 25, it would have been very different. ❞

Volume displacements

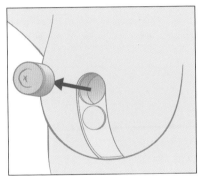
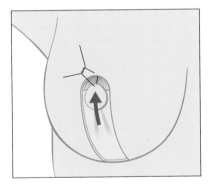
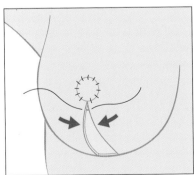
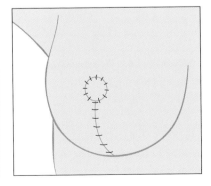

Excision of tumour under the nipple

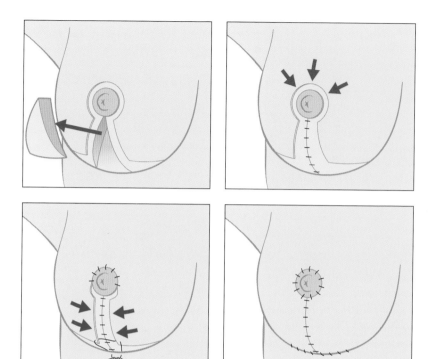

Excision of tumour in the lower part of the breast

Complications of surgery

These techniques are more complex than a straightforward 'lumpec-tomy' or partial mastectomy. As a result, complications are a little more common than after lumpectomy alone. Following volume replace-ment, the blood supply of the flap may fail occasionally. When this happens the flap may have be removed and discarded. Following volume displacement, very occasionally the blood supply to the breast tissue isn't good enough. When this happens further tissue has to be removed and this may lead to a poor result.

Making your choice

One of the most difficult things about breast cancer is having to wait for the diagnosis to be confirmed and then being asked to make decisions about the type of surgery you prefer to have done.

> " I had to wait two weeks for the biopsy results and they were the worst two weeks out of the whole thing. I did get upset then. I already had a gut feeling that it was cancer because my mum's sister was roughly my age when she was diagnosed and she died of it after it had come back in her bones. My dad's sister died of breast cancer when I was very tiny. I have always known since I was a kid that I would get it. It wasn't really a big shock when they told me. My friend who was with me was more shocked. As soon as I was told that it was cancer, I thought that I had to get on with it. There was no point in crying and being miserable. "

It's often helpful to meet or talk to other women who have faced similar choices to you. Your breast team should explain your options, and help you with pictures and printed information about the different techniques. It's important you ask about anything you don't understand and if you're unhappy about advice you've received, you're entitled to ask for a second opinion.

> " I was 74 at the time I was told that I needed to have a mastectomy. I have always had a horror of mastectomy. I did not want to have one and looked for other solutions that would stop that. I can't believe that I was the only woman feeling like that.
>
> I wonder whether there was an ageist thing with me. When I asked the first doctor in the clinic about reconstruction, he told me that we could talk about that later. I thought that I should have known about that at the time. I felt that they thought it wasn't worth bothering with reconstruction at my age.
>
> Of course reconstruction has been worth doing at my age. After having a second opinion, my reconstruction was quite simple, but I felt that I was denied the initial discussion because of my age. Other people should not be put off if they want to pursue it.
>
> When looking for solutions that avoided mastectomy, the second surgeon suggested removing just the disease in the one breast and then reducing the size of the other breast to balance them at the same time. I was very happy with that. Having surgery on the unaffected breast didn't worry me. I thought that it was a brilliant and happy solution. "

***Appearance after volume displacement for a tumour in the lower part
of the right breast (the left breast has been reduced in size to match)***

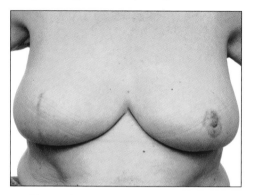 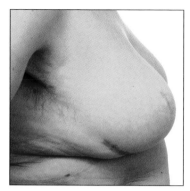

Front view   *Side view*

If your surgeon thinks you'll need radiotherapy after the operation,
it's likely you'll be advised to avoid having a reconstruction with an
implant. You may be encouraged to consider delaying reconstruction
altogether until after all your treatment has finished, or to think about
having an autologous LD, TRAM flap or partial reconstruction, as
none of these techniques involve the use of an implant.

" The surgeon then said I could either have a mastectomy and after
the chemotherapy and radiotherapy was finished, I could have
the breast reconstructed, or I could have a latissimus dorsi
miniflap reconstruction. With this, sometimes after the
radiotherapy the muscle shrinks and looks a bit odd. I was told
that it was up to me. They are both long operations but the full
reconstruction takes longer. I was offered a TRAM flap because I
was advised not to have an implant and then have radiotherapy.
However, I did meet other women who had implants at
radiotherapy. I decided straight away which one I was going to
have. I thought that a really long operation was silly and I
couldn't cope at the time with the thought of losing my whole
breast. I thought that I would rather keep as much of me as
possible. The possible risk of the shape changing after
radiotherapy didn't enter into it. I just didn't want to wake up
without a breast there. I had a partner at the time and he was
very supportive and upset but didn't take part in the decision-

making. What got me was how upset everyone else was. I felt fine but couldn't handle everyone else. I talked about it with my partner, friends and my brother and sister-in-law. I just wanted to get it done as quickly as possible.

I saw the breast care nurse and she showed me pictures. They didn't really make a difference because I had made my decision.

Don't be stampeded, take your time when deciding what to have done. People get scared when they have cancer and think that it must be dealt with immediately. I thought that it had been going for some time, so I should see what the options were. Even if a partial reconstruction had not been an option, I would have probably tried the full reconstruction. I have no regrets at all. Even though my breasts were a better shape before the treatment, the main thing is that they are still there.

What will it be like soon after the surgery?

Having a partial mastectomy and reconstruction is a smaller operation than a full mastectomy and reconstruction, but a bigger procedure than having a mastectomy without any reconstruction at all. Most patients are pleasantly surprised to find that it's not very painful when they wake up. This is because powerful painkillers such as morphine are often used, and the amount can be selected by you the patient by pressing a button. This delivers a small dose into your blood stream every time you need it. In many hospitals, the anaesthetist will use a technique to deaden the nerves around the reconstruction using local anaesthetic, which can last for twenty-four to forty-eight hours.

I can't remember pain when I woke up, although I was on morphine to control it. I had three quite large scars, one on my back, one in my armpit and one below the breast.

The one on my back was fine. I had no trouble from that. The one under my arm was the most painful. All the drips and drains made it harder to go the loo.

I looked at my breast while I was still in the hospital. I felt fine. I didn't care after I knew that I had not lost the breast. I kept my nipple. I did show my partner and that was all right. He wasn't offended by it.

I was in hospital for a week and by the time that I went home could do most things apart from lifting. I was washing and dressing. I went and stayed with my brother and was looked after.

My arm movement was all right straight away. I was given exercises by the physiotherapist and I did them. I go to the gym twice a week at least and if I miss it, for example because of going on holiday, it gets stiff and pulls under the arm. I went back to the gym throughout the radiotherapy four or five times a week. I was trying to lose weight before going on holiday. I just did a gentle programme that was devised by the trainer at the gym after I told him what I had done. It really helped. I was very unfit, having not been active during chemotherapy and radiotherapy.

I was in hospital for two nights. There were teething problems with the healing and at first I clutched myself when I turned over in bed and my breasts were a bit sore for a while. You mustn't be too depressed when it doesn't go right immediately because it will in the end. I found it helpful to be warned that it could take time to heal. I was very tired in the beginning but if you are sensible, you pace yourself.

What about long-term recovery?

If you've had volume replacement with a miniflap, you may be aware of numbness over your back where the muscle was taken from and experience some tightness around your chest. You may also notice some 'jumping' of the muscle in your breast, particularly if you move suddenly or sneeze. You'll find that within a few months of surgery most of the new sensations will settle down.

My armpit and the top of my arm are still numb. I can feel where the muscle was moved but not above it. I have sensation to the upper outer part of the breast. The sensation has slightly improved and my back is numb. It is annoying but that is all. Very occasionally, when I cough, the muscle in the reconstructed breast jumps slightly. It doesn't really bother me.

It is a year since the operation and I can do anything. I do know that my left arm is weaker and I have not got quite the movement when raising my arm above my head, but I have got a full range of movement, apart from that. I don't have central locking in my car and I would not now lean right across the car to use the arm on the reconstructed side to undo the door lock. I would walk round instead. That is the only thing that I have changed.

Initially, the reconstructed breast matched the other one well but I have lost two stone since then. That means that the reconstructed breast has stayed the same size and the other breast has shrunk a bit. The side of the breast under the arm, where the muscle has been brought through is fuller than the other side. I was warned that if I lost or put on weight, the breasts might not match.

I was told that with the TRAM flap, the reconstruction would lose or gain weight with me, whereas it wouldn't with the miniflap. The difference is not that noticeable. Nobody else has noticed. I now wear non-wired bras, which are quite comfortable. I can't run in the gym because the muscle in the breast is too heavy and painful. I was advised to wear a bra for support a lot of the time, which was helpful. It also helped in bed.

I finished the radiotherapy three months ago and I think that it is still slightly affecting the breast. 〞

If you've had volume displacement with reduction in the size of both breasts, you may notice numbness in the lower parts of the breast and around your nipples.

One of the great benefits of partial mastectomy and reconstruction using either volume replacement or displacement is that your breast feels pretty normal and looks pretty normal. And, unlike full mastectomy and reconstruction, your breast will feel like part of you, rather than something that has been made to look like a breast but doesn't feel to you like the real thing.

〝 At the beginning, the breast was a bit numb. The back of the arm and around the scar felt as though I had pins and needles. This probably went on for a year to eighteen months. I could cope with that as my activities were not affected by it. It was just a strange feeling when I touched it. Even now, five years later, when I have done things which I shouldn't have done, for example, heavy lifting, I feel the muscle tightening where the scar is in my armpit but it lasts for a couple of seconds and is gone. I don't remember having much numbness in my back.

"

7 Reconstruction of the nipple and areola

- **Nipple reconstruction can have a big effect on body image.**

- **It can make a major difference to the appearance of your breast.**

- **There are many different types of nipple reconstruction.**

- **The choice is influenced by the amount of projection you require.**

- **Most nipples are made longer than the opposite side, to allow for shrinkage.**

- **Tattooing is optional, and often needs to be repeated after twelve to twenty-four months.**

Your nipple, also known as the nipple–areola complex (NAC), includes both the nipple and the surrounding pigmented area of skin, called the areola. Nipples are usually projectile, although some can be inverted or flat, even with stimulation. The little bumps on your areola are called Montgomery's tubercles – these extra-large 'goose bumps' are glands that secrete a waxy fluid to moisturise and protect your areola and nipple. Your areola also contains hair follicles, and hairs can be quite prominent in this area. There are about fifteen to twenty-five 'lactiferous' ducts that pass from the glandular breast tissue through your nipple. These ducts transport milk to your nipple, as well as providing projection. The colour, size and texture of the nipple is highly variable across ethnic groups and in different individuals, although the NAC is usually darker than the surrounding skin.

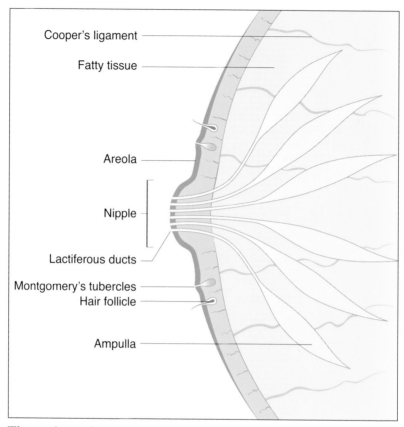

The nipple–areola complex (cross-section)

The NAC is integral to the overall appearance of your breast, a feminine symbol of nurturing and eroticism. NAC reconstruction is usually the final step of breast reconstruction following mastectomy. Women with other conditions, such as congenital or developmental abnormalities of the nipple, burn deformities, and complications following surgery including breast reduction, can also benefit from NAC reconstruction.

> Although the reconstructed breast was a natural shape, I was left with a flat circle of skin where the nipple should have been. Whenever I looked at it, I was reminded of what I'd had. I thought that having had such a good reconstruction, it would be a shame not to complete the process.

> " Having been pleased with the breast reconstruction, I felt inclined to have the nipple reconstructed to rid myself of all the artificial attachments (adhesive silicone prosthesis). "

Reconstruction of the NAC can have a big effect on your body image and overall quality of life. Making an NAC that matches the position, size, shape, projection and colour of the other side can make a big difference to the appearance of the reconstructed breast and to the overall result. These are currently achievable goals, but creating a new nipple that can become erect and has full sensation are goals for the future. There are many different ways that your NAC can be reconstructed. We'll take a look at the most commonly used techniques.

Principles and techniques

It's normal to have your nipple reconstructed as a day-case under local anaesthesia. There are some general principles that are common to all techniques:

- NAC reconstruction is usually postponed until your breast reconstruction has settled down. This is usually about three months after your operation. A few surgeons will reconstruct your breast and your NAC at the same time.

- When your new NAC is being reconstructed, your own NAC serves as a template. Both you and the surgeon should find time together to plan the position of your new NAC. Various techniques can be helpful when deciding on the best place, including using the sticky dot usually used for making heart traces, or a sticking plaster. You can stick the dot in the best position for you, while looking in the mirror.

- If you're having both sides reconstructed your surgeon will rely on certain well known anatomical landmarks to choose the location of your NACs. In general, they will be located at the apex or most projecting point of your new breast mounds.

- To begin with, your new nipple will be almost twice as long as the one you've lost. This will allow for the shrinkage, which is inevitable, particularly in the first three months.

> “ I had dressings on the nipple and it healed up in a few weeks. It did not affect my normal activities. ”

> “ In my case, it took almost six months to get the nipples right. At first the nipples looked a dreadful sight while they were healing. They were made long to allow for shrinkage. Most of the shrinkage takes place in the first few weeks and months. They are perfect now and look so real. ”

It's easier to understand NAC reconstruction if we look at the operation in two steps – first the nipple, and then the areola.

Nipple reconstruction

Over the last forty years or so, many different techniques have been used for nipple reconstruction. These techniques include using the original nipple, using the nipple from the remaining breast, using grafts of skin and cartilage from the ear, as well as tattooing alone. Some of these techniques are no longer used.

Currently, local 'flaps' provide the most reliable techniques. These use local tissue that is rearranged to create a 'bump'. This local tissue may well be the skin 'island' from your breast reconstruction, in other words the skin from your tummy or your back. The skin over your reconstructed breast is numb and because of this, nipple reconstruction is usually a painless experience. There are many different ways of creating a bump and we will discuss the best current and most commonly used techniques. The best techniques are simple, giving long-term projection, and provide a good blood supply. Healing is good and there is minimal scarring in the site from which the skin has been borrowed.

Your surgeon will often make your new nipple larger than the one on the other side because the new nipple will shrink in size over the first year or so. Nipples made from skin borrowed from the back tend to be firmer than those made from tummy skin – reflecting the much thicker skin we have on our backs. Swelling and scabbing around a new nipple is very common in the first two weeks, but this will settle down naturally as healing takes place.

The skate flap

The skate flap was introduced in 1984 and became the most popular technique for nipple reconstruction. Two thin skin flaps, shaped like the wings of a skate fish, wrap around the central fatty core and create a prominent nipple. This is a good choice for a large projectile nipple. The skate flap sometimes requires a skin graft to close the residual defect.

The skate flap

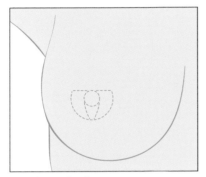

Marking the flaps

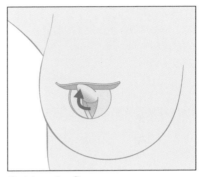

Raising the flaps

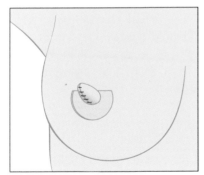

Forming the nipple

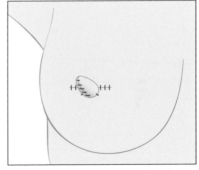

Closing the defect and the final result

If your surgeon decides to use a skin graft, this will also create a new areola around the nipple. The skin can be 'harvested' from different parts of the body. Common areas include the groin, the inside of the thigh or the end of the scar where your flap was taken from. It can even be taken from your other breast if you are having reduction of your other breast to match at the same time.

The CV flap

The CV flap was introduced in 1998. It is made from a central core with a hat and two thinner arms that wrap around it, producing a less pointed shape than the skate flap.

The CV flap

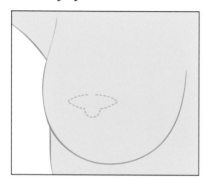

Marking the flaps

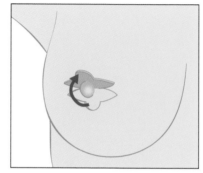

Raising the flaps

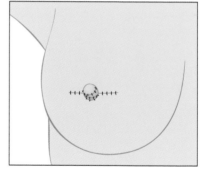

Forming the nipple

Closing the defect and the final result

This type of flap leaves a smaller gap in the surrounding skin than the skate flap. This means that it's usually unnecessary to use a skin graft and a new areola can be made by tattooing the surrounding skin to hide the scar if required. Your surgeon will often advise waiting a few months before doing this to allow the scar to mature and settle down.

The arrow flap

The arrow flap was introduced in 2003 and is a modification of the CV flap. Essentially it is very similar to the CV flap except that the two arms dovetail in the shape of an arrow rather than lying side-by-side, in the case of the CV flap.

The arrow flap (modification of the CV flap)

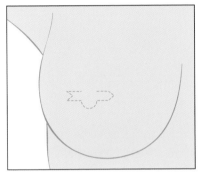

Marking the flaps

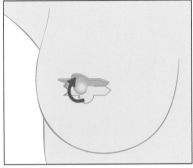

Raising the flaps

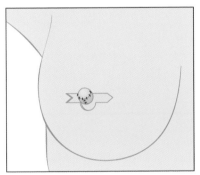

Forming the nipple

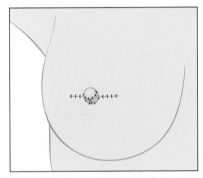

Closing the defect and the final result

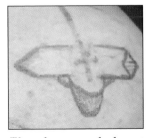

Flaps drawn on the breast

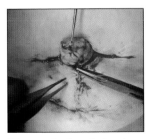

Flaps raised and closed

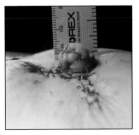

Nipple height

121

Attempts have been made to provide long-term projection of the nipple by using firm material during the reconstruction of the nipple. Cartilage grafts can be used to augment the nipple reconstruction, and cartilage can be removed from your rib at the time of certain kinds of breast reconstruction, such as DIEP or TRAM flap reconstructions. It can then be 'banked' under the skin of your breast or your abdominal wall for use at a later date.

Areola reconstruction

Reconstruction of the areola can be achieved very successfully by tattoo alone or by skin grafting. 'Nipple and areola sharing' methods are rarely used today. In this method, the normal unaffected areola is reduced in order to create a new areola on the reconstructed breast. Donor site scarring and potential damage to milk ducts and breast-feeding, as well as to the erogenous structure, have made this technique unpopular. Skin grafting is a commonly used technique for areola reconstruction. The upper inner thigh is a popular site for taking a full thickness skin graft, as skin from this area is more pigmented than breast skin. Other sites include skin from the labia and from behind the ear. These are not so popular as patients find them less acceptable.

NAC reconstruction using full thickness skin graft from the upper thigh

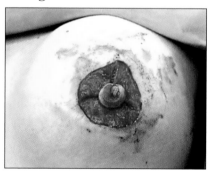 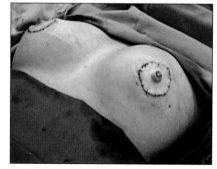

Ready for graft   *Full thickness grafts in place*

Tattooing

The quality of pigments available for medical tattooing has improved greatly over the last fifteen years, giving a more natural and less 'painted on' appearance. Tattooing can be used independently for areola reconstruction (the reconstructed nipple is also tattooed a darker shade than the areola) or as a final 'touch-up' technique to achieve the best colour match and symmetry. Tattooing is generally done six to twelve weeks after nipple reconstruction to allow your wounds to heal and your nipple to contract down. Some surgeons prefer to have the tattoos done before nipple reconstruction. The advantages of tattooing are the lack of need for a donor site and extremely realistic results. It can be done on an outpatient basis, is quick to perform, and risks such as allergies are very low. The disadvantages of tattooing are that the pigments fade with time and therefore secondary touch-ups are not uncommon. The technique of tattooing requires training and experience to achieve good results. Rarely, overcorrection with the tattoo may persist.

Stages of tattooing: the patient had a delayed DIEP breast reconstruction followed by nipple reconstruction alone (the normal nipple is small)

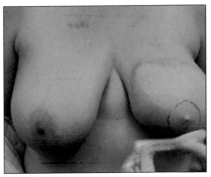

Marking the areola

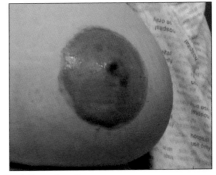

Applying the pigment

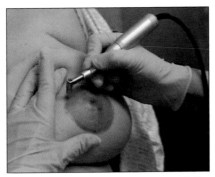

Tattooing (no anaesthesia needed)

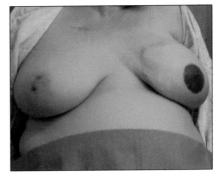

At the end of tattooing

Results

The following pictures show a selection of postoperative results. These are average results and not necessarily a selection of the best. Nipple reconstruction is often carried out three to six months after breast reconstruction, using a technique such as the CV flap (described above) followed by areola tattooing some six to twelve weeks later.

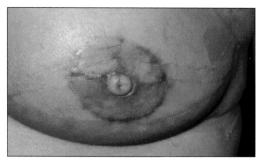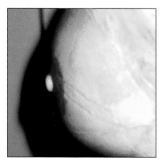

Latissimus dorsi (LD) with implant reconstruction and nipple reconstruction with full thickness grafts

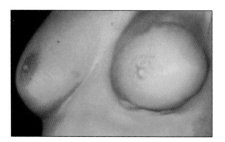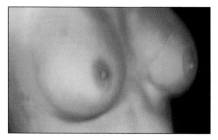

Left delayed DIEP breast reconstruction with faded NAC reconstruction requiring top-up tattoo (the areola was a tattoo only)

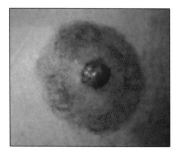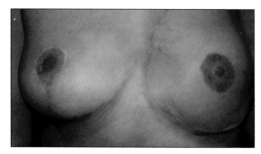

Left delayed DIEP flap breast reconstruction and NAC reconstruction with right-sided reduction (the areola is a tattoo only)

" I was not so happy with the match of the new nipple but after having the colour tattooed on, I felt much happier. "

" The reconstructed nipple did have some colour but as it settled down over a period of time, it became patchy. I had it tattooed to make it a better colour match. I think that it was worth it. You can live without it but it is important for the sake of your appearance. "

" Although I was very pleased with the nipple reconstruction as it was, I decided to have the nipple colour tattooed on as well. I had been completely undressed once or twice in the female showers at the swimming pool and just felt slightly conscious that one side was coloured and the other was not. The colour was not uniform all over. I have been told that it will fade. I shall leave it and see how it goes but know that I can have it coloured again in the future. "

" I did have a nipple reconstruction, which initially was thoroughly disappointing because it was not a good shape and it turned white when it healed. However, it was still better than having no nipple. I took the breast care nurse's advice and had the nipple tattooed and it looks much better now. The size and colour of the area matches the other breast and I am glad that it has been done. "

Complications

Complications of NAC reconstruction are rare, but they need to be discussed. They include wound infection and wound breakdown, and there may be partial or complete nipple loss if the blood supply to your nipple is poor. This may be due to the design of the flaps, or sometimes where radiotherapy or smoking has affected the blood supply of the skin. A common complication is loss in the projection of your nipple. This is usually acceptable, but correction can be achieved using local tissue, cartilage or commercial fillers if required. Complications of areola reconstruction include fading of the tattoo and, rarely, a tattoo that is too dark. Top-up tattooing to correct fading is a simple procedure. Complications of areola reconstruction when your surgeon has used a skin graft include wound infection and poor graft 'take'. This happens when the skin doesn't pick up a good blood supply from its new position on the breast and some of the skin dies away. This can lead to loss of part of the graft, or occasionally the whole graft.

Special situations

You have the greatest risk of complications after NAC reconstruction if you have your breast reconstructed using an implant alone or have had radiotherapy given to the tissues being used for the NAC reconstruction. Simple techniques are the best in this situation, as the wounds are slower to heal and are more likely to break down.

Conclusions and the future

Modern techniques can rebuild a very life-like NAC with little discomfort and a high degree of patient satisfaction. In the future, new techniques will focus on creating a more realistic nipple, possibly using innovative tissue engineering techniques.

" I am very pleased with the nipple and it is nice to feel complete. I went abroad a couple of months ago and it was lovely to be able to put on and take off a swimsuit like everybody else. "

" Since having the tattoo done, I am now able to shower in the communal changing room at the swimming baths without worrying about people looking. The colour of the tattooed nipple has gradually faded but I know that I could have that redone if I had the time. "

" The breast looks better with a nipple because there is no longer a blind piece of skin in the centre and it had some interest to it. That makes a lot of difference and I think that it makes me feel more confident. I would have been fine without it but it is rather nice to have it. "

" The nipple has made a difference to the appearance of the breast. I am not as conscious as I used to be when in a communal changing room. I am more embarrassed for other people than me. I am ready to go topless on the beach and can wear a T-shirt without a bra. "

What can you do if you want a nipple but no more surgery?

For some people, the thought of another operation, however minor, in order to have a nipple reconstructed may not be appealing. Another option to consider would be to use a prosthetic (false) nipple, which is attached to the breast using a special adhesive. These nipples come in two different forms:

- Nipples made in silicone by the companies who make breast prostheses. They are available in several sizes and colours.

- Individually made nipples that are made to match the patient's own nipple shape and colour. These are usually produced by technicians in conjunction with Breast Units. The advantage of these is that they can look very realistic.

Sometimes is can be helpful to try using the silicone nipples for a while to see how you get on with them if you are unsure about the surgical options. The best way to find out about how to get these is through your Breast Unit. They will be able to tell you what is available.

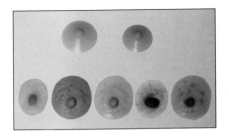

Custom-made and individual nipples (upper row: commercially available nipples; lower row: nipples made for individual patients)

8 Surgery on your other breast

- Operations on your normal breast are done to prevent cancer or to match your reconstructed breast.

- It's important to decide what size you want to be before having your breast reconstructed.

- Your surgeon can then plan to enlarge, reduce or lift your normal breast.

- These operations are usually done after you've recovered from your reconstruction.

- You should weigh up the risks and the benefits of these procedures before going ahead.

When facing mastectomy, many women worry about their other, normal breast. They may feel that the unaffected breast is particularly important and precious, or they may fear that breast cancer will affect that breast as well. They may even ask their surgeon to remove their normal breast at the same time as their diseased breast. There are four different kinds of surgery that can be carried out on your normal breast. These should be considered by you and your surgical team when planning your overall treatment. Your options include risk-reducing mastectomy, breast lift, breast reduction or breast enlargement.

Risk-reducing mastectomy

In some women a strong family history of breast cancer increases their risk of developing cancer in the other breast. Your surgeon and an expert in breast cancer genetics will be able to work out your own risk of developing cancer in your normal breast based on your family history. If this risk is high then a risk-reducing mastectomy, with or without reconstruction of your other breast, may be a very sensible option. To some extent this can depend on the stage of the cancer in your affected breast. For example, a woman with an excellent prognosis early breast cancer but who has a high risk of cancer developing on the other side because of her family history would be a prime candidate for a risk-reducing mastectomy.

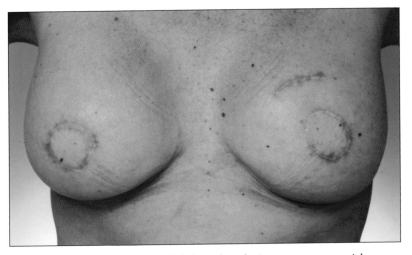

Left mastectomy for cancer and right risk-reducing mastectomy with immediate reconstruction

Deciding whether to have a risk-reducing removal and reconstruction of your normal breast will affect the type of breast reconstruction chosen for both sides. Most women will decide they don't want a risk-reducing mastectomy on the normal side. If this is what you decide, your natural breast will be used as a template for your new breast and nipple reconstruction following removal of your diseased breast. Your surgeon will try to match your normal breast as closely as possible by shaping your reconstructed breast. Occasionally, it may be difficult or impossible to match the natural breast, and then surgery to lift, reduce or enlarge it may be needed to achieve symmetry. Unfortunately, any surgery on your natural breast will involve scarring. Complications such as haematoma, infection and difficulties with healing can occur, as well as loss of sensation.

If you have a mastectomy and immediate reconstruction this will give your surgeon the best chance of matching the opposite side. It's much more difficult to get a good match following delayed reconstruction. Much depends on a woman's bra size and cup size. These can only be taken as a guide – the actual bra size and cup volume differ between manufacturers. A woman with an A, B or C cup breast who has a reconstruction using an implant may well achieve a breast of sufficient volume. But it's difficult to get a natural 'ptosis' or droop using implants or expanders alone (see p. 33). So if you're in this situation the natural breast may need to be lifted to match the other side. These techniques can be especially beneficial for women who can't find a suitable bra or clothing because their breasts are so unbalanced following reconstruction.

Breast lift

A breast lift is known as a 'mastopexy'. The volume of your natural breast may be sufficient in a bra, but when your bra is removed there is an excess of skin that allows your breast to sag and drop below the level of the reconstructed side. Your nipple will be in a lower position as well, and the whole breast looks lopsided. The mastopexy operation moves your nipple and areola upwards on the natural breast mound

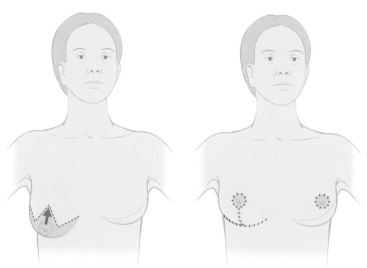

Right mastopexy for symmetry after left breast reconstruction (left nipple reconstruction at the same time)

and removes skin in order to tighten your breast and elevate the central 'dome'. The scars needed for this will always extend around your nipple and areola and often pass straight down towards the bottom of your breast. There is sometimes another scar which lies in the crease where the breast joins the chest wall – the 'inframammary fold'. A mastopexy is particularly helpful if you're flat in the upper part of your breast. Having a breast lift won't increase your breast volume though. It will simply reorganise the volume that's already there, moving it into a different position. Complications can occur after mastopexy – in particular, some nipple sensation may be lost.

Breast reduction

If you have large natural breasts, a breast reduction combined with a breast lift may be the best option. This is known as a reduction mammoplasty. Women with large heavy breasts may feel quite relieved to have their new breasts reconstructed to a smaller size, and then to have a reduction of their natural breast to match. The breast tissue that's removed during your reduction will be examined by your pathologist and checked for any abnormality. It's also good practice to carry out a mammogram on your natural breast before undertaking reduction surgery.

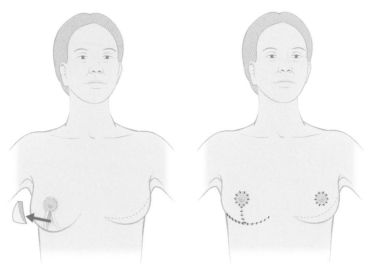

Right breast reduction for symmetry after left breast reconstruction (left nipple reconstruction at the same time)

You should discuss all the complications of a reduction mammoplasty with your surgeon, who should explain how your breast will look after it's healed. Your final size will depend on what you want and what can physically be achieved on your reconstructed side. Scars following breast reduction are usually anchor-shaped, similar to those after some types of mastopexy. They run around the areola and there may be a shorter vertical scar passing down into your inframammary fold. A short vertical scar like this will often be 'crimped up' by your surgeon in order to try to eliminate the need for a scar running along your inframammary fold. Following this kind of surgery, your scars and the shape of your breast will take three to six months to settle.

During a reduction mammoplasty, your surgeons will remove excess breast tissue from the lower and central parts of your breast, lifting the nipple and areola to the new position on a higher, smaller breast mound. The nipple is kept alive through the normal tissue lying behind it. Very occasionally, the nipple is lost because of a poor blood supply. Fortunately, this happens very rarely – about one in every two-hundred cases. There may be some numbness of your nipple after the procedure, but usually this isn't permanent.

It's important that your reconstructed and reduced breasts look symmetrical at the end of the operation. Inevitably, you'll have some bruising and swelling after the surgery, and the lower pole of your reduced breast (the part below your nipple) may look quite flattened for the first few weeks. But as long as healing occurs normally and you don't develop any complications, you can expect reasonable symmetry in the medium and long term. Your surgeon can find it difficult to judge exactly how much tissue needs to be taken away if this operation is done at the same time as your breast reconstruction. For this reason, many surgeons will delay the reduction of your natural breast until a later date, perhaps combining this with reconstruction of the new nipple and areola on your reconstructed side.

66 Because my bra cup size was a D, I opted to have the reconstructed breast made smaller by two cup sizes and have the other side reduced later to match it. I was not worried about the operation but about the fact that someone was going to operate on me and make me look different. I was amazed about how emotionally I thought about the operation.

I am usually a busy energetic person with work and walking my dog every morning for 45 minutes. After the reconstruction, it was three months before I could walk down to the beach and back again, which was a steep walk of a mile and a half. I was amazed how grotty I felt. My brain was still cotton wool for the first six weeks. I thought that I would go back to work after three months but it was six months before I went back part-time. I am sure that I would have been able to do full-time work with a bit of a struggle but it was exhausting. It was only after eight months that I started to get any oomph back.

I had the other breast reduced later to match the reconstructed one, which was super. Luckily my breasts were so saggy that I had enough skin to make an areola and a nipple on the other side at the same time. That operation was not at all uncomfortable afterwards. It healed within ten days. I was very keen to have this done, and in particular have the injection port removed because it was uncomfortable and my bra always seemed to get stuck under or over it.

My husband says that my appearance now is absolutely fine. He is just so pleased for me that I can wear a bikini top for sailing and I can dig on my allotment. I have not had to change any of my clothes. It is now a year since the operation and I can do anything.

I wasn't expecting to be so shocked or the fact that I felt 'got at' after the operation. I don't think about it now but it went on until I had the other breast adjusted. I was very conscious of being lop-sided, although people did try to reassure me that I didn't look lop-sided. I think that reconstruction is so great compared to having a space and having to keep a false breast there. I like the fact that I do not have to think about it at all now.

It was a real shock to be told that I needed a mastectomy. After having a second opinion, I was quite happy with the idea. We talked through the options, taking into account my work in catering, which involved a lot of heavy lifting. At the time, I intended to go back to that afterwards. I also played golf. It was decided that I should have a mastectomy and an immediate latissimus dorsi reconstruction with a tissue expander. Due to my breast size, I was also to have the other breast reduced at the same time. This is a good idea because you don't notice it and it just heals while the reconstructed breast is being sorted out.

It is over two years since the operation and I feel fine about my appearance. It's not too great when I am stripped off but when you are 60, it's not too great anyway. I don't feel conscious of it at all when I am dressed and I don't think that anyone notices, even though my breasts are not quite level. My husband is quite happy about it because the bottom line is that I am still here and that is the important thing as far as he is concerned.

The big bonus about reconstruction is that if you do a lot of swimming, or when you go on holiday, you don't have to think about a swimming costume. I still wear the same style that I wore before the surgery. After reconstruction, you do want to wear bras that are nice. You have a cleavage and can take the neckline of clothes down a bit. You want to feel attractive again and it can be done. The fact that the breasts are different only matters between yourself and your partner. As long as the relationship is working, then it is not a problem. You do need help with underwear but don't need to go to a specialist. Any lingerie department that does fitting should also talk to you and fit you.

"

"
After the tissue expansion was completed, my reconstructed breast was much smaller than the other side. I was told that this was because I had radiotherapy and the skin would not stretch so well. I was offered an operation on the other breast to make it smaller and lift it up to match the reconstruction. I thought about it and decided to go ahead but my husband did not want me to because he said that it was not necessary. I have decided not to go ahead at the moment. It can be difficult to find bras and clothes to suit my shape. Buying bras from the mastectomy companies can be expensive. I adapt my bras myself with shoulder pads to balance the shape.

"

Breast enlargement

Sometimes women want to have their new breast reconstructed to a larger size than that of their natural breasts. If you're in this situation, your surgeon will need to enlarge or 'augment' your normal breast to match using an implant. There's a wide range of implants available that come in a variety of shapes and sizes. Implants may be dome-shaped or round, or anatomically shaped, like half pears or teardrops. Most modern implants are made either from silicone 'cohesive' gel, injectable salt solution (saline) or a combination of both. There are two different types of design. 'Fixed' volume implants have a permanent volume that can't be adjusted, whereas 'tissue expanders' allow your surgeon to adjust their volume after the operation (see p. 31 for full details).

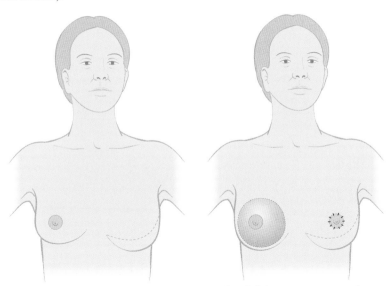

Right breast augmentation for symmetry after left breast reconstruction (left nipple reconstruction at the same time)

Augmentation of your breast is usually a straightforward procedure with few complications. An implant needs to be used to perform your augmentation, and in time it may need to be exchanged for a new implant. Implants can also become enclosed with a hard shell of tissue called a 'capsule'. Surgery may be required to remove this capsule if it becomes painful or causes distortion of your breast. Breakdown and rupture of modern implants are rare. The new 'cohesive' gel implants don't contain liquid silicone and have thick shells, making the likelihood of rupture very low. It's worth bearing in mind that they can affect the sensitivity of mammograms, and you should inform your radiographer so that she can use a special technique that is helpful in women with implants. Implants and expanders can be inserted through small incisions. These are usually in your inframammary fold or in your armpit. Some numbness of your natural breast may follow augmentation, but implants can be removed and replaced with day surgery if reshaping of the breast is needed at a later date.

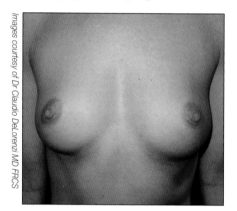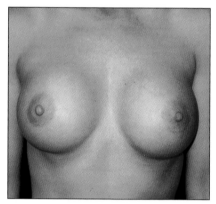

Images courtesy of Dr Claudio DeLorenzi MD FRCS

Appearance after augmentation of both breasts

Conclusions

These are the main techniques that are used by surgeons to achieve symmetry after your breast reconstruction. It's important to realise that, like your left and right feet, your left and right breast are never the exact mirror image of each other. There's always some natural asymmetry, and even after a breast reconstruction and balancing operation there will always be differences between the two sides. The pursuit of perfection can result in unnecessary surgery for little gain, and can expose you to unnecessary complications and risks.

9 Possible complications after breast reconstruction

- **Complications are less common in fit and healthy women.**

- **Complications include those that can happen after any operation, as well as those that depend on the technique you choose.**

- **Most complications aren't life-threatening and can be treated effectively with good overall outcome.**

- **You should ask your surgeon to explain your risks of developing complications before you sign your consent form.**

You're thinking seriously about having a reconstruction, but you want to know about the risks of this kind of surgery. What can go wrong? How bad can it be and how can complications be avoided?

All of these questions should be answered before you give your consent for surgery. You'll be asked to sign a form that should summarise exactly what's going to be done. It should also give a brief summary of the complications that can happen. Doctors are expected to let you know about serious or frequently occurring mishaps. It would be very long-winded and quite frightening to list every possible complication, so you must ask your team to explain any particular complications you are worried about. For example, if your work or sports activities involve pushing your shoulders backwards (for example, golf, cross-country skiing, vacuuming), this may be slightly impaired by a latissimus dorsi (LD) procedure and you may decide to choose a different type of reconstruction.

General health

Your surgeon will take into account your occupation, lifestyle and social responsibilities when advising about suitable types of reconstruction for you. They'll also want to know if you are fit enough for major surgery, because both the anaesthetic and the operation carry risks. Generally, the fitter you are, the better the outcome. You're less likely to have complications if you are slim, young, physically active, don't smoke and don't have any significant health problems. But we're not all perfect specimens and there are factors than can increase the risks of your surgery. Obesity is associated with an increased chance of chest infection, clots in the leg, wound infection and wound breakdown. Smoking is associated with chest infection, wound infection and problems with the blood supply to your flap. At the very worst, this could mean that the flap won't survive and will have to be removed.

Lung problems

When you've had a general anaesthetic you're more prone to developing plugs of mucus, which can block part of your lungs. This is because it can be difficult and uncomfortable to move around and take deep breaths to clear your airways. Your nurse or your physiotherapist can help you to take a deep breath and cough to get rid of any blockage, but this can be difficult after major surgery because it's uncomfortable in the early days. Pain relief, deep-breathing exercises and keeping well hydrated are all very important after surgery, and can help to prevent any blocked parts of your lungs from getting infected. This is important, as if any infection isn't properly treated it can occasionally lead to pneumonia.

Thrombosis (blood clots)

Clots in the leg are more likely after operations because your blood gets stickier following surgery – the blood pools in your calves as you lie still on the operating table and because you become dehydrated. Steps can be taken to prevent clots forming with injections to thin the blood, compression stockings, calf squeezers in theatre and other manoeuvres. You can also help yourself by paddling your feet up and down every fifteen minutes or so, and by shifting about in bed. Try to move about as much as you can and ask the nurses to help you to sit out of bed as soon as you're feeling strong enough. Drink plenty of water, as the atmosphere in hospital tends to be dry.

Infection

Any surgical wound can become infected, but infection around a breast implant can be a major problem. Implants are made of inert synthetic material that the body's defence mechanism can't penetrate. If bacteria get into a wound during surgery or on the ward, they can settle round an implant and are almost impossible to eradicate. If this happens the implant may have to be removed, although it is usually possible to replace it with a new one when the infection has settled down. Infections are usually caused by the bacteria that live on your own skin getting into tissue that has been traumatised by surgery. You are more likely to get an infection if your immune system is weakened, for example if you take steroid medication or have diabetes.

If the blood supply to the tissue is poor because of atheroma (clogging of the arteries) or because of smoking, which causes spasm of the small blood vessels, infections can get hold. Infection may be no more than redness or soreness of the wound, but it can progress to cellulitis (a spreading infection of the skin) or it can form an abscess. Usually no more than a few extra days of dressing and a course of antibiotics is all that is needed to deal with the infection. Very occasionally, the infection can lead to blood poisoning (septicaemia), which can turn into a very serious, life-threatening condition unless it's treated early and effectively.

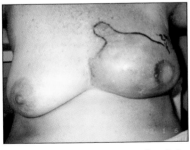 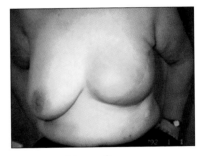

Infections in two patients after left mastectomy and immediate reconstruction

Scars

There will always be scars after surgery. If these are carefully placed and stitched up well, the ultimate scar will be nearly invisible, but it can take up to two years for scars to settle and for the redness to disappear. Some people are more prone to these raised, thickened and red scars, known as 'hypertrophic' scars. A very small number of people will develop 'keloid' scars that continue to thicken and don't settle down without treatment. Younger women and those with darker skins are more likely to be affected. Continued pressure on the wound with tape or silicone gel may help to reduce the likelihood of these thickened scars developing. Most surgeons now use an 'invisible mend' type of suture (sub-cuticular stitches), but clips and removable stitches can give good results if they are removed early.

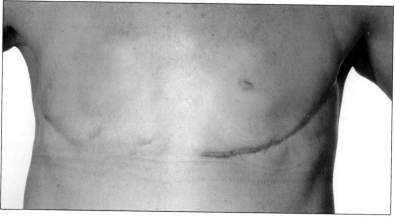

Scars after bilateral mastectomy (right side normal scar, left side hypertrophic scar)

Bruising and haematoma

Drains are used to collect fluid from the operation site immediately after surgery. They also collect blood. Great care is taken during surgery to prevent any bleeding – coordinated teamwork of all the theatre staff is essential. Electrical cautery (which heats the blood vessels) is used to seal the smaller vessels, and clips and ties are used to seal the larger vessels. Bleeding after an operation is very common and usually shows itself as bruising. Occasionally, bruising can be quite extensive, but if this happens it will disappear in a week or two. Larger collections of blood are known as haematomas. These are usually left to clear of their own accord if they are not rapidly enlarging or causing pain or putting pressure on the overlying skin or implant. Occasionally, haematomas become infected and will need to be emptied or evacuated. This is usually done under a general anaesthetic in theatre. Smaller haematomas can usually be treated by sucking the fluid out with a needle and syringe. If you develop a large haematoma that continues to get bigger, you may need to return to the operating room. This can happen within hours of the initial surgery finishing – usually because a large artery has 'popped' – or a few days after surgery when a vein starts to leak. Sometimes the bleeding is enough for a blood transfusion to be needed. It is essential that you let the surgeon know if there is any reason why you cannot have a blood transfusion before you go ahead with your reconstruction. If a transfusion is likely and your reconstruction is not urgent, you can arrange to pre-donate some of your own blood or boost your iron levels with tablets or injections before your surgery.

Bruising after breast surgery

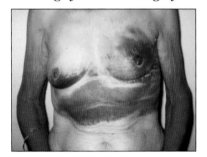

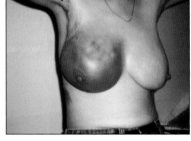

Extensive   *Localised*

Seromas

Seromas are collections of fluid that have accumulated in spaces left behind after surgery. They are not dangerous and are expected to some degree after any operation. Sometimes the fluid builds up pressure and becomes uncomfortable. If this happens under your arm, it may be difficult for you to put your arm down by your side. Fluid often builds up in the gap if you have had the latissimus dorsi (LD) muscle taken away from your back (the 'donor' site). This can feel like walking around with a 'hot water bottle' on your back, as the fluid sloshes around when you move about. A build-up of fluid may be uncomfortable and it can occasionally become infected. Seromas can also interfere with the planning of other treatments, such as radiotherapy and chemotherapy. Your surgical team will usually 'aspirate' (draw away) the fluid if it's uncomfortable or if you're waiting to have other treatments. This should be completely painless because the area is numb and you shouldn't feel the needle. Sometimes this will need to be repeated several times until the fluid goes away. Care will be taken to avoid introducing infection into the seroma by using a sterile technique and by reducing the number of times the seroma is drained.

Seromas in donor site after LD breast reconstruction

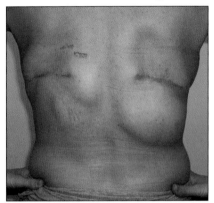 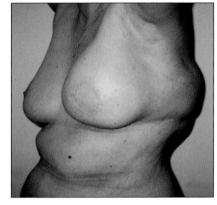

Both sides   *Left side*

The fluid can be drained away with a needle and syringe, but if the fluid is not bothering you it will be left alone to reduce the risk of introducing infection. Some surgeons use techniques that may reduce fluid collecting in the tissues, such as closing the gap with stitches. Seromas are less likely to be troublesome after delayed reconstruction or flaps involving your tummy.

Sometimes seromas persist for many months. If this happens, the tissue around them becomes hardened and this 'bag of fluid' may have to be removed by surgery.

Pain

Part of the anaesthetist's job while you are asleep is to ensure you feel as little pain as possible after the operation. Most breast operations are surprisingly painless, but with reconstruction, because there's been more surgery, there's a greater need for pain relief. The anaesthetist will discuss pain relief with you before the operation. A local anaesthetic is often used to deaden the nerves in the wound as well as the nerves coming out of the spine that supply the area. It's quite likely that you will have a little button to press to control any pain when you wake up. This delivers a small dose of a very powerful painkiller straight into your bloodstream (patient-controlled analgesia – PCA). If it's been used, it will be replaced by a 'cocktail' of painkillers, including anti-inflammatory drugs, within twelve to twenty-four hours of your operation. You may need to keep taking painkillers for three to six weeks after reconstructive surgery.

Your reconstructed breast and the upper part of your arm will normally feel numb when you wake up. This is because the nerves that supply the skin of your breast are cut away as the breast is being removed. The nerves to your breast never really recover and most of your breast will always feel numb. The nerves supplying the skin on your arm will often recover, particularly if your surgeon has taken care to preserve them. They are usually stretched during the operation and may take three or four months to recover. The skin on the inside of your arm near your armpit may feel strange while the nerves are re-covering – burning, tingling and 'pins and needles' are common sensations that will eventually settle down. If your nipple has been pre-served, it will almost certainly be numb and will not become erect.

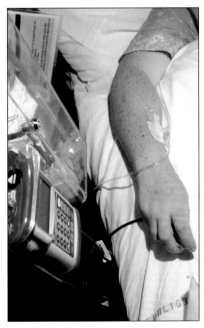

Patient using a PCA device

Lymphoedema after reconstruction

Lymphoedema means swelling of your tissues. It happens because fluid from your lymphatic system gets trapped and cannot escape. Your lymphatic system is a network of fine vessels that help to defend you against infection. After breast surgery this fluid can build up and affect your breast or your arm. It can happen after any kind of surgery to the glands in your armpit and it's no more likely to happen after recon-struction than after surgery without reconstruction. The chances of it happening will depend on how much surgery has to be done on your glands, and whether or not you need to have radiotherapy to your armpit.

The lymph glands in your armpit normally act as 'nets' to capture and destroy particles that could do harm if they got into your bloodstream. Cancer cells are close enough to normal cells to fool the lymph glands, so cancer cells can settle and grow in these glands. It's usually the first sign that the cancer is on the move if the glands are involved. That's why it's important to remove the lymph glands draining the breast to treat the cancer and give you an idea of how well you're going to do in the future.

Lymphoedema of the breast

Sometimes removing the lymph glands under your arm (your 'axilla') will block the drainage of lymph fluid, which then builds up in the tissues of the reconstructed breast. This can produce heaviness and swelling of the breast skin, which then looks similar to the skin of an orange, so it is often called 'peau d'orange'. Gentle regular twice daily massage can help redirect the fluid away from the tissues towards the lymph drainage areas. This problem usually settles down gradually.

Lymphoedema of the arm

Performing surgery in your axilla can also block the flow of lymph from your arm. This is not usually a problem immediately after surgery, but can occur many months or years later. Even a small amount of surgery in the axilla can trigger off lymphoedema. Removing glands as part of the cancer surgery as well as finding the

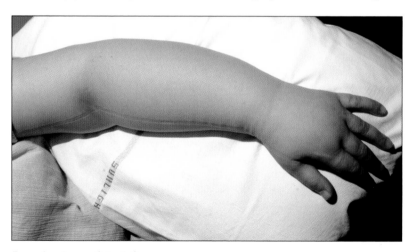

Lymphoedema of the left arm

blood supply to a latissimus dorsi flap can affect the lymph channels from the arm. About one in twenty women who have glands removed from the axilla will eventually develop some swelling of the arm. A small cut or graze or infection anywhere on the arm or hand can set it off. You will be given written information before your operation explaining how to avoid these problems and how to treat them.

Lymphoedema may not affect the whole arm – it may involve the hand, the forearm, or the upper part of the arm. In its early stages the fluid can be treated by compression or massage. It can be prevented from getting worse by wearing a compression sleeve. If the fluid remains for any length of time it can act as an irritant and cause scarring within the tissues. This makes the tissues harden and makes it much more difficult to treat. Radiotherapy to the armpit increases the chances of lymphoedema following surgery. It's very uncommon to give radiotherapy to the armpit after surgery to clear all the lymph glands because up to one in every four women treated in this way will get lymphoedema.

Sentinel node biopsy

Although your doctors need to know whether your cancer has spread to your lymph glands, it may not be necessary to remove very many glands to do this. Two techniques to remove a small number of glands have been developed. Both techniques cause lymphoedema in less than one in a hundred women. The first technique takes at least four glands from the armpit for analysis and is accurate at predicting problems. The second technique, the 'sentinel node' biopsy, is a more refined approach using a blue dye and a small injection of radioactivity to find the lymph gland most likely to have cancer in it. The dose of radio-activity is tiny (less than living in Aberdeen or Cornwall for a year) and between one and three glands are usually removed. Not all hospitals are able to provide this service at present and it is not suitable for all women. Further surgery is usually required if these techniques show cancer in the glands that have been removed.

10 Will my reconstruction be affected by my breast cancer treatment?

- **The key aim of your treatment is to prevent your cancer from coming back.**

- **Your overall treatment will not be delayed if you choose reconstruction.**

- **Radiotherapy can have an adverse effect on your reconstruction, especially if an implant has been used.**

- **You may be advised to delay breast reconstruction if your team thinks that you're going to need to have radiotherapy after your surgery.**

When you've had your operation, the pathologists will examine your tissues carefully and they will look for a number of features that will tell them much more about your tumour. This will help you, together with your doctors, to decide which treatment is best for you and to explain the risks of the cancer coming back, as well to assess your overall chances of a good outcome. Depending on what this examination shows, you may be advised to have further treatment to cut down any chance of the cancer returning and to improve your overall outlook. These additional treatments include radiotherapy, chemotherapy, hormonal treatments and antibody treatments – all of which are given to fight cancer.

Your doctors will advise you which treatments are best for your individual case, depending on what kind of tumour you've developed and what kind of benefit you're likely to gain. Some patients don't need any further treatment at all, some need all of these treatments and some need a selection. Your cancer specialist (oncologist) will be able to give you an idea of the benefits of each treatment and will help you to make the decision.

Radiotherapy and breast reconstruction

Your team will advise you to have radiotherapy if there's a real risk of the cancer returning in the area where your breast was removed. Although chemotherapy may be effective in reducing this risk a little further, it's not as effective as radiotherapy. Radiotherapy will reduce the risk of cancer returning in the region of your surgery by about two-thirds, and it's also a routine part of your treatment if you've only had part of your breast removed and reconstructed (see p. 102). But it isn't needed for eight in ten women who've had a full mastectomy, and is isn't needed at all if you've already had a mastectomy and are having a reconstruction later on. Radiotherapy can have an adverse effect on the appearance, texture and comfort of your new breast.

The early effects of radiotherapy

The early effects of radiotherapy are the same in patients who've had a mastectomy whether or not they've had a reconstruction. The same number of patients may experience dryness and reddening of the skin during their radiotherapy treatment.

Longer term effects of radiotherapy

Much is known and understood about the changes caused by radiotherapy in the breasts that haven't been reconstructed. Although initially the breast tissue seems normal and the breasts appear symmetrical, there will be changes that continue for many years. A number of studies have looked for these changes in women who've had breast reconstruction. There isn't a lot of information because not many women have had this kind of treatment in the past and they haven't been followed up for long enough to give us a full picture. But early results suggest that the timing of radiotherapy as well as the type of reconstruction could be important factors.

Timing of breast reconstruction and radiotherapy

Reconstruction may be carried out either at the time of initial surgery – immediate reconstruction – or after all additional treatments such as chemotherapy and radiotherapy have been given – delayed recon-struction. Immediate reconstruction has many advantages but if radiotherapy is required, the risk of scarring and loss of softness of the reconstructed breast is greater than if the reconstruction is delayed until after radiation treatment has been completed. These risks are also higher in patients who have radiotherapy immediately after surgery, rather than several months later after chemotherapy has been completed.

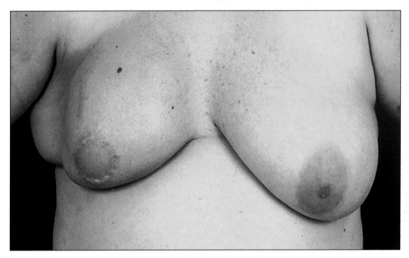

Severe distortion of the reconstructed right breast after radiotherapy

Radiotherapy with breast implants

When an implant alone has been used for the reconstruction, there's a real risk that the breast will become hard, painful and distorted, giving a cosmetic result that is less than satisfactory. This is because of firm scar tissue forming around the implant. Overall, when radiotherapy has been used after reconstruction using an implant, a third of patients rate their cosmetic result as good, a third rate it as satisfactory and a third rate their appearance as poor. Because of these effects, if you're likely to need radiotherapy after surgery your surgeon is likely to advise you to delay reconstruction until you've finished your radiotherapy or to consider a different technique that doesn't involve the use of an implant.

> " After the tissue expansion was completed, my reconstructed breast was much smaller than the other side. I was told that this was because I had radiotherapy and the skin would not stretch so well. I was offered an operation on the other breast to make it smaller and lift it up to match the reconstruction. "

Radiotherapy and breast reconstruction with your own tissue

Radiotherapy may also cause problems following reconstruction using all your own tissue, including the autologous LD and the TRAM flap techniques (see pp. 44 and 73). But the chances of a poor result appear to be much less than following reconstruction with implants alone. Again, the risks are higher when radiotherapy is carried out immediately after surgery rather than when it is delayed or carried out before surgery. It may lead to hard patches in your new breast ('fat necrosis'), as well as some shrinkage and loss of movement of your breast. Nevertheless, about eight of ten patients feel that the cosmetic appearance of their new breast after TRAM flap reconstruction and radiotherapy is excellent or good.

Other things that may add to the effects of radiotherapy

There are also some aspects of your general health and lifestyle that can add to the effects of radiotherapy. If you smoke, suffer from high blood pressure or you're overweight, the effects of radiotherapy and the complications of your surgery may be increased.

Chemotherapy and breast reconstruction

Your doctors may advise you to have chemotherapy after your surgery, once samples of your tissues have been examined by the pathologists. This treatment is usually started about four weeks following your operation or when your wounds have healed. Even if you develop complications, it's unusual for your chemotherapy to be delayed for more than a week or two. There is no evidence that this affects the success of your treatment, or that chemotherapy causes any harm to your reconstructed breast.

Hormonal treatments and breast reconstruction

Your team may recommend hormonal treatments, and again there is nothing to suggest this will have any adverse effect on your reconstruction.

Monoclonal antibodies and breast reconstruction

In the future, we're going to see more doctors using 'monoclonal antibodies' against various cancers. These treatments, including Herceptin®, target and kill off cancer cells. It's too soon to know about and understand the side effects of these complicated treatments and whether they have any effect on the breast that has been reconstructed or irradiated.

Summary

In summary, if you're given radiotherapy before surgery, immediately after surgery or after chemotherapy, it can change the tissues to make them feel firmer and look less natural. These changes seem to be less common after reconstruction using your own tissues. All the same, most patients are happy with the cosmetic outcome and where there's a real risk, radiotherapy helps to stop the cancer returning in the breast. It's important to realise that once you've had radiotherapy it has an effect that continues throughout your life. That's good in one sense because if you're at risk it will help to stop your cancer coming back in your breast. But it may gradually change your shape, preventing the enlargement and 'dropping down' of the breast that happens naturally as you get older. So your team will weigh up the risks and benefits of these treatments with you before advising you whether you should have radiotherapy after your surgery.

11

'Risk-reducing' mastectomy and reconstruction for high genetic risk

- **Genetic testing may be done if you have a relative with a faulty gene.**

- **You'll be given specialist advice about having this test and dealing with the results.**

- **You can choose from several options if you're found to have a faulty gene.**

- **If you're considering surgery, you'll be seen by a range of experts before making a decision to go ahead.**

The location of the first major high-risk breast cancer gene within the human genetic fingerprint was discovered in 1990 on a chromosome called 'chromosome 17'. The gene was called BRCA1 (BReast CAncer 1). It was found to be faulty particularly in families in which many young women developed breast cancer, as well as in those who developed ovarian cancer, although it took another four years for the full genetic code for BRCA1 to be worked out. The BRCA2 gene was identified in 1995. This was discovered through selection of families with male as well as female breast cancer patients for study, although many families with the faults or 'mutations' that produce the BRCA2 gene do not include men who have developed breast cancer. Ovarian cancer occurs with both genes, but is more common in women with BRCA1 than with BRCA2 genes.

Genetic testing of families with a very striking history of breast (and often ovarian) cancer was offered from the mid 1990s. Initially, the families who were offered this testing were those who had taken part in the research to find the genes. This was rapidly introduced into the

NHS, although often with patchy provision of services. As technology has improved, the speed of testing for mutations in these large genes has improved. In a small proportion of families with many cases of breast cancer, a mutation in either the BRCA1 or BRCA2 gene can be identified that explains the strong family history. The very few women who have a mutation in either gene have a high risk of developing breast cancer. Up to eight out of ten of these women develop breast cancer, and the average age at diagnosis is below 50 years. But it's important to recognise that only 20–30% of families with multiple breast cancer cases are explained by these two high-risk genes. There are many other genes that probably increase breast cancer risk. Some are extremely rare high-risk genes and many are lower risk genes. At the moment, they aren't any more useful than the family history alone in helping your doctors to estimate your risk of breast cancer, but they may become useful as research moves forward.

You may be referred to the Regional Specialist Genetics Service if you're worried about a strong history of breast cancer and perhaps ovarian cancer in your family. This is the starting point for assessing whether it will be helpful to test your genes. Your local breast cancer service may also be able to make an initial assessment of your genetic risk and provide you with advice about surveillance, but detailed genetic testing is offered only through your Regional Specialist Genetics Service. A clinical geneticist can review information about your family tree and types of cancers that your family members have had to find out if genetic testing is likely to be useful in your case. The genetics service can also give advice about your long-term cancer risks and can discuss options for dealing with this. You can then formulate an action plan that will be agreed with your breast cancer screening and treatment teams.

If you have a strong family history of breast cancer, you often feel very vulnerable. Past experience (such as the long-term survival or death of a close relative) can naturally influence your concerns about your own risk of breast cancer. If a strong history of breast cancer or breast and ovarian cancer is identified in your family, the first step in evaluating your genetic risk is to get as many of the medical details about the cancers in your family members as possible to help your geneticist decide whether genetic testing is going to be helpful for you or not. Next it's necessary to contact someone from your family who's had breast or ovarian cancer to find out if they are willing to provide a blood sample for genetic testing. This is because any one family will have its own often unique mutation in the gene, if one is present at all, and it could be anywhere throughout the entire gene. The DNA, which is your 'genetic fingerprint', is then examined in fine detail. This is a bit like proofreading a large textbook looking for a tiny spelling mistake! If a fault isn't found in either gene, this almost entirely rules out a high-risk gene as an explanation for your strong family history, but it doesn't rule out the involvement of genetic factors that haven't yet been discovered. When a genetic test is possible it can be very helpful. On one hand, it may show that you haven't inherited the faulty BRCA1 or BRCA2 gene that's causing the high risk of breast cancer in your family, and you can be reassured that your risk is similar to the risk of breast cancer in the general population. On the other hand, if genetic testing shows that you do carry a high-risk gene, there are a number of options to help you cope with that risk.

Your options in general terms if your testing shows you have a high genetic risk include:

- watchful waiting – this includes breast awareness, mammography and other breast-imaging, such as magnetic resonance imaging (MRI)

- risk-reducing measures using medication, such as tamoxifen

- risk-reducing measures using surgery, such as removal of both your breasts (bilateral risk-reducing mastectomies) and/or removal of both of your ovaries and fallopian tubes.

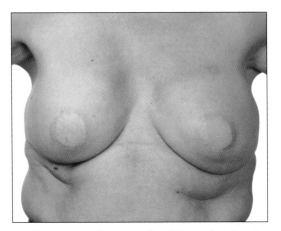 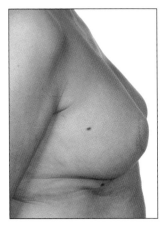

Front and side views after bilateral risk-reducing mastectomy and immediate latissimus dorsi reconstruction

" My grandmother had ovarian cancer and my mother had breast cancer, as did my sister. My middle sister was also diagnosed with the BRCA2 gene and has recently undergone preventative surgery and reconstruction. I knew that I was a high-risk candidate given my family history, and I wanted to be proactive in mitigating against that risk.

Before I had the test, I visited the genetics clinic and discussed the issue with the staff. They were extremely supportive and wanted to ensure that I fully understood the implications of having the test, and what it would mean to me if it came back positive.

'A journey of 1000 miles begins with the first step' and I felt that this was the first and hardest step to take. I did not believe that I would not have the gene; I just did not feel that lucky! I knew that if I started on this journey, then I had to be sure about what my intentions were if I had one of the BRCA genes. I was not going to have the test and then not do anything about it. I had watched my mother die, and my sister fight cancer. I did not want to go through that myself.

We discussed how the test was done, what the lab would be looking for. As my sister had already had the test, the lab would just look for the particular strain that had been discovered in her. It was explained to me how long the results might take, and we also talked about what my options were if I had the gene. Most importantly for me, and this might not be the case for everyone, we talked about what I thought the result would be. I needed to talk to someone who understood my fear of not knowing but also the fear of knowing. Although I felt prepared for the result to be positive – I did think I would have one of the BRCA genes, it was an enormous shock when the nurse told me, just to hear those words spoken out loud. I was understandably upset, and needed time to absorb it. Even if you expect bad news, it is still a shocker when it arrives. "

" At least six members of my family, including my grandmother and mum, have had breast cancer. Another aunt had ovarian cancer. My mum died when I was 24.

I wasn't keen to be tested to start with, I suppose because I was quite young – in my 20s. I didn't feel that it was a problem for me at that time. As I turned 30 and had my own family, I became concerned that if I did have the gene, then it could become a problem for me. I then made the decision to have the gene test.

I was seen in the Genetics Clinic a few times before I was tested and I was made aware of screening that was available to me. It was very reassuring to be given so much information. It made the decision much easier for me to make. I was not under any pressure to go ahead, just well supported. I made the decision to be tested. My husband was very supportive and felt that I was doing the right thing by being tested.

I felt disappointed when the results of the gene test showed that I had a breast cancer gene. I had hoped that I wouldn't have it. That was partly because of my daughter as well. I just wanted it to end and stop with me. I have been surrounded by people with breast cancer since I was young. It wasn't a huge surprise, just a bit sad really. I knew before I was tested that if the result was positive I would have surgery.

"
I was upset when I was told that I had a breast cancer gene, even though I knew it was possible because of my family history. It was final then. However, I needed to know.
"

If you are someone who carries a breast cancer gene and you do develop breast cancer, it's often found early and can be treated in the same way as breast cancer in anyone else, with conservation of your breast. But if you have a strong genetic risk it means that you have a higher chance of developing breast cancer at some stage in the future – either in the same breast or in your other breast. It's also very likely that even an early breast cancer would need additional treatment, including chemotherapy and radiotherapy. Some women, knowing they have inherited a family gene, decide they wish to have their diseased breast and their other healthy breast removed as a preventative procedure. Once breast cancer is diagnosed, the priority is to treat the cancer and to reduce any threat of the cancer returning.

Any surgery to reduce the risk of developing breast cancer in your other breast can be considered once you've recovered from the treatment of your cancer. This doesn't have to be decided until all your treatment has been completed and you've made a full recovery.

For some women who carry a high-risk breast cancer gene, the decision to have both breasts removed (bilateral mastectomy) before cancer is diagnosed seems simple, for others it's very difficult but may feel like the only option, and for yet others it's just not an acceptable option. Each individual needs to be provided with full information on more than one occasion. In general, if you're looking for help to make up your mind you'll have plenty of opportunities to discuss different strategies with experts. You'll be encouraged to explore and discuss your options, and to come to your own decision about managing your breast cancer risk.

If you're thinking about bilateral mastectomy to reduce your risk, you'll be given the opportunity to see a range of experts. These include the clinical genetics team, a breast surgeon, a plastic surgeon (some surgeons are expert in breast and plastic surgery), a breast care nurse and a clinical psychologist or specialist counsellor with expertise in this area. The psychological and psychosexual effects of this type of surgery need careful consideration by you and also by your partner. Attendance of partners at these sessions can be very helpful, and is strongly encouraged.

> " Although I decided before undergoing genetic testing that if the result was positive, I would have preventative surgery, discussing mastectomies and breast reconstructions when I was fit and healthy was one of the hardest things to come to terms with. I felt like a fraud, taking medical help away from people who were actually sick. This was the issue that I spent the most time talking about to the breast care team. Whilst I understood that taking a preventive step in the first place would hopefully save all the subsequent treatment if I had developed cancer, it still took some time to become comfortable with the concept.
>
> I was put in touch with a lady who had been through a similar situation. It was particularly helpful talking to someone who knew what I was going through. My husband and I also went for psychometric testing prior to the operation. This gave us the opportunity to talk through intimate issues as a couple and also individually with a counsellor.

After the operation I felt numb – very bruised and battered. I looked at myself in a mirror lying down on the first day. I was by myself and I just needed to see how I looked. The second day, I stood in front of the mirror for a long time; it took some getting used to, but I needed to get to grips with the reality of how I now looked physically. I also knew that once the bruising and swelling had gone down, things would look a lot better.

I am an extremely fit person. I was back at the gym within seven weeks of the operation. I started swimming and underwent a series of hydrotherapy treatments, which were amazingly beneficial.

I had almost seven months off work in the end. I had originally planned to go back to work after four months but I had some emotional difficulties, particularly with the way I looked, and in the end, I did not go back to work for another three months.

During the recovery period, I would advise people to do only as much as they feel like doing. If they are tired, lie down. If they start to feel emotional and blue, seek help early.

I am happy with my overall look. I take more care over my appearance now; it is very important for me to look feminine and attractive, and I am sure that is linked to losing my breasts. My husband thinks I look good, probably fitter than I did before! Sexually he misses my nipples and we don't make love face to face as much; he won't say that the way my breasts look are an issue, but I am sure that he misses the feel of a natural breast. He is just too considerate to tell me, and would not want to upset me.

I have found it hard to come to terms with the loss of an essential part of me that makes me a woman. My breasts do not feel the way they did before; they are not soft or pliable and there is no sensation, but I would do it all again. The relief that I am not going to wake up one morning and find a lump is tangible.

Overall, the experience, give or take a few events, was exactly as I imagined and had been described to me. I felt I was as prepared as I could be for the operation. Emotionally you have no idea how the operation is going to impact on you. I am a strong person, and believed that I would be able to cope with it. I did, but it took a while; you will feel and look differently as a woman – this experience has changed my outlook on many things. ”

" I knew before I was tested that if the result was positive I would have surgery. My husband felt that I was doing the right thing to have the surgery once I found out that I had the gene. In his mind I had been tested, I had the breast cancer gene and I had a problem. The only solution was to have the surgery and he gave me all the support that I needed.

I was 35, with three children aged four years, three years, and nine months. Contemplating major surgery when I was fit and healthy was a solution to a problem in my mind; it was something that had to be done and I was keen to get on with it so that I could move forward.

I have a cousin who really didn't want to have mastectomies and breast reconstructions and it took her a long time to come to the decision. It was the only option that she had but she still didn't want to have it done. Now, she is glad that she did go ahead and she doesn't regret it.

When I first woke up I felt as though I had been hit by a bus. I was quite shocked at how battered I felt. It is hard to prepare for that because I have never had anything done that has made me feel like that. I was in hospital for six days. I did feel that I made progress as time went on. I didn't really feel strong enough to go back to the house with three toddlers but actually, when I got home the family were very good and it worked. I was discharged with six drains still in. I carried them about with me. My children thought that they were wonderful and were very curious. They were removed at home later.

I needed a lot of help when I got home, especially with the children. I wanted to do a lot of things myself and got frustrated because I couldn't do them. I did more things gradually as I improved.

Having both breasts removed and surgically reconstructed was a major thing to go through and I would advise others to make sure that they have lots of support. You have to explain to people that you are going to be very tired and restricted. Even after three or four weeks, you may look better and have your drains out but you still feel very sore, particularly on the back. The tiredness persists and you have to make sure that you get lots of rest. It is two or three months out of your life when you are going to feel battered and bruised and frustrated that you can't do the things you normally do but it is a small price to pay and an easier option than having breast cancer and going through the treatment that goes with it.

Eighteen months after having both breasts removed and reconstructed I am fully able to cope with a demanding family life and hard physical work as well. It has been worth going through all of this to lessen my chances of getting breast cancer. The only thing left from the operation is that the scar across my back is tight but that is better than having breast cancer. It doesn't show with swimming costumes. I didn't expect to be pleased with the result of the surgery but I am. "

" After the mastectomies and reconstructions, I was upset in a way because although my breasts had been reconstructed, I felt as though part of me had gone. That feeling improved and I did not grieve for my breasts later.

I developed an infection in the wound and that delayed everything. The infection lasted from September to January, when the implant was removed. I then had six months without the implant. The time without the implant wasn't good but you have to keep going. I had support. My family were great, my husband was good. I felt awful having to go back into hospital to have the implants put back again. It was the thought of having to go through all that again. I had to have them done again though because I wouldn't give up. I got there in the end. I didn't want to do without breasts.

I am pleased with the look of my breasts now. I don't think that they have changed much over time. I think that they have dropped a bit and there are a few creases here and there. I am confident in most clothes. It feels a lot thicker under my arms. Apart from that, it doesn't bother me.

There were bad times during the infection but as far as my appearance is concerned now, I don't regret that at all. I only have to think about what my mum went through and that justifies it. "

Here's a husband's viewpoint:

" To me, once we knew that my wife had a breast cancer gene, deciding to have surgery was a simple logical decision. Why wouldn't you do it? If anyone gets breast cancer, they have the operation done. All of a sudden, due to cancer research, the doctors are able to tell you whether you have the risk before you get the cancer.

My concerns weren't about me but about how it would affect my wife emotionally. It was an unknown to me. I never discussed the operation with anybody. I always felt that it was never my business to do that.

You could get stressed out beyond belief, but all a man should tell himself when his wife is having that surgery is to think how you would feel if she was having the surgery for cancer. I was grateful to be in the position of having a wife who was not trying to get rid of breast cancer with the chance that it could come back. We knew that there was an 80% chance that she would get breast cancer but we knew that with surgery, there was no more risk of getting breast cancer than the person sitting next to us.

It was an anxious lead up to the time of and during the surgery but the second it was done, particularly for my wife, there was a great anxiety lifted. The healing took place quite quickly. The anxiety that we would otherwise live with for the rest of our lives had disappeared. To my mind, the plastic surgery that my wife had is amazing.

I would advise any husband or partner to take a deep breath for a few weeks while it is all going on and hold on tight and then thank everyone afterwards. It is easy for the bloke to give advice because we don't have to have it ourselves, but if I was told that I would get testicular cancer unless I had surgery done, why wouldn't I have it done? I would be an idiot not to. I didn't have to persuade my wife to have the surgery done. She made her own mind up anyway. "

12 Getting ready for your breast reconstruction

- **Take time to find out about your reconstruction, and don't be afraid to ask questions before you go into hospital.**

- **Your team will be able to answer all the important questions about how you are going to look and feel, and how long it's going to take you to recover from surgery.**

- **Your recovery will depend on the type of operation, as well as your own health and motivation.**

Once you've decided whether breast reconstruction is for you and have chosen what type of breast reconstruction to have, being well prepared for the surgery will help you cope better and recover more quickly afterwards. Many women who have to come to terms with their diagnosis and other possible treatments at the same time as understanding breast reconstruction, feel as if there's too little time to take everything in. While it may be important to you to have the surgery as soon as possible, it's vital for your overall recovery that you fully understand the implications and possible complications before you have your operation.

Either way, having to go into hospital to have an operation can be very traumatic, and research suggests that the more suitable the information you have, the less you'll suffer from uncertainty, anxiety and possible distress (see p. 180). You can then plan ahead with your family and home arrangements, as well as your work commitments, so that you have plenty of time to recover until you're fully fit. Your partner or children may also have questions about your recovery that they would like answers to.

Talking to your Breast Team

You're likely to have plenty of practical questions to ask about your operation, and the specialist nurses in your Breast Unit are the best people to talk to. Your nurse may be either your breast care nurse or a nurse working with the plastic surgeon who's looking after you. It can be very helpful to write down your questions beforehand, as well as having another person with you to listen to the conversation and support you. It's worthwhile remembering that any question you need an answer to is important, particularly if the answer helps to relieve any of your fears or anxieties. Your specialist nurse can spend time with you and your family explaining the surgery as well as the practical implications in simple terms, so that you fully understand what's involved. She'll answer your questions and listen to your fears, and will also encourage you to explore your feelings while offering a sympathetic shoulder to cry on if necessary. It's also quite a good idea for you to ask to see your surgeon again if there are further issues that need to be explained.

Some questions it's helpful to clarify before your operation

What will I look like and how will the breast feel?

The best way to find out about the scars is to ask to see photographs, and to talk to another patient who has had a similar operation. Remember that another patient's experience may not be exactly the same as yours. Sensation in your reconstructed breast, your arm and other areas affected by the surgery can differ from person to person. Ask what you can expect from your operation.

What sort of dressings and stitches will I have?

You should find out what to expect and who will care for your dressings once you leave hospital. You may well have drainage tubes coming out beside your scars to drain any extra fluid away to help the tissues to heal. These should not restrict your movements very much, and some patients go home while these are still in place. Most wounds are closed these days using stitches that are hidden under the skin and don't need to be removed.

Will the operation be painful?

Immediately following your operation it's possible that your operation site and arm movements will be uncomfortable, sore or painful. It's usual to be given regular painkillers, often using a system that allows you to control your pain relief yourself by pushing a button. This is called 'patient controlled analgesia' or 'PCA' and it will be reduced as the discomfort settles and you begin to recover (see p. 143).

How long will I be in hospital and what will I be able to do afterwards?

This can be very variable, depending on the type of operation. Check how long your team expect you to stay in hospital and what care you're going to need once you get home. Ask about the 'do's and don'ts' when you get home, and for how long you need to be careful.

How long will I take to recover?

Again, this varies, depending on your operation, other treatments and your normal lifestyle. Take time to talk this through with your specialists. Some types of breast reconstruction are major operations and the recovery period can be quite long, so try to be realistic about this from the outset.

How long will I be off work for?

You'll need to know from your team how much time you're going to need off work. But remember to tell your employers that this could change, depending on how quickly you recover. It's helpful to review this from time to time during your recovery.

When will I be able to drive again?

This will depend on the type of breast reconstruction you've had. It may take longer to be confident driving if you've had abdominal surgery, but again, check with your team.

Will I have to go back to outpatients regularly?

Check on the number of expected outpatient visits after your operation. This is particularly useful information if you're unable to drive yourself and need to get help with lifts from your friends and family.

What sort of bras and clothes should I bring into hospital?

Some surgeons like their patients to wear specific supportive bras after breast reconstruction. Check whether this is the case for you and if so, whether they are provided by the hospital. If your surgeon doesn't have any special recommendations, get advice from your specialist nurses about the type of bra to wear afterwards and find out if you need to take it into hospital with you. There are different options immediately after your operation, and later on.

> " I was advised to get a sports bra by the hospital to wear after the reconstruction. What I actually wore was a vest-type top with a bit of support, rather than a bra. I found that the bra strap irritated. Vest tops with part support were very good. "

> " I wear sports bras for comfort but know that I can wear prettier ones for other occasions. I have bought a bra with no wire in and that is quite nice and does give me support. I can't just go and buy any bra but have to try them on. The ones that I think are nice don't always fit properly. The reconstructed breast is a better shape than the other one. "

> " The one thing that I do not like is the fact that I cannot wear the type of bras that I used to wear, which were underwired and dainty. Whilst I have found bras that are comfortable, they are not as feminine. I went to Eloise [a shop specialising in bras and accessories designed to be worn after breast surgery; see p. 219 for further details] for underwear and found them extremely helpful. I have bought their lingerie ever since. I wish that there was a bra that was wider under the arm. You don't feel discomfort at the front, it is at the side. "

> " Because the area that has been operated on is sensitive, a lot of bra fabrics are itchy. Certain laces were difficult and cotton was better. I think that it took about a year after the operation to get back to normal bras. I now change in a communal changing room and once I have my bra on, there is no difference, apart from the radiotherapy scarring. "

It can often be easier to wear pyjamas or a buttoned nightdress immediately after surgery, in case your arm movement is restricted or to make regular inspection of the surgery easier.

Will I need to do exercises after my operation?

Ask about the arrangements to help you with your physiotherapy (see p. 169). It's really necessary to practise these exercises because they'll help you get your arm movement back and speed recovery.

Will I need to have further operations to complete the reconstruction?

Breast reconstruction is rarely completed in one operation, so do ask your surgeons how many operations you're likely to need. If it's necessary to have more surgery to complete your reconstruction, it can be difficult to get used to the idea of going back into hospital if you're not expecting it.

Following surgery, you'll see that your breast shape has been altered. This may take you some time to get used to. You may find it helpful to look at the scars while still in hospital and then to get used to gently touching the changed area, by carefully massaging cream into the healed scars. Some women also find it helpful to show others their new breast as soon as possible, but these are very personal choices.

When you first look at your breast after reconstruction, it will probably look swollen and bruised. Any operation takes time to settle down and heal. If you're having tissue expansion after your surgery, don't forget that when you first look at your reconstructed breast it may be smaller or larger when you compare it with your normal breast, and it's likely to be a different shape.

> 66 Because of the tissue expansion, when I first looked at my new breast, my chest looked massive and I couldn't escape it. I wanted to forget about it but it seemed so much there. You have to keep positive because it doesn't look good to begin with. It helps to think back to the photographs of the end results and know that you will get there. 99

Regardless of what type of surgery you have, you'll probably get tired easily to begin with. It's important to take things easily and you'll need to avoid strenuous exercise for several weeks after surgery. As you recover and the wounds heal, you'll gradually be able to resume normal activity.

> " When I first woke up from my latissimus dorsi breast reconstruction, I felt that it was behind me and I was on the road to recovery. I could do everything when I went home but it took quite a while to get my strength back. I wouldn't say that it is an easy operation because it was six months before I could sleep on my side. That was a minor thing, though. I had nearly six weeks off work. "

During the recovery period everyone is affected differently. There may well be a time when you experience a range of varied emotions and you may need to be gentle with yourself, particularly when you feel tired. You might well have good and bad days during this time but the number of good days will increase as you recover.

Here's an account from a 34-year-old woman who had a latissimus dorsi breast reconstruction. Her two small children were a priority in her recovery:

> " It was decided that I would have a latissimus dorsi breast reconstruction with a tissue expander at the same time as the mastectomy. I did get upset in the first few days afterwards because I couldn't see the light at the end of the tunnel. You have to be prepared for the incapacity afterwards. I felt that it was important to get moving as quickly as possible.
>
> I couldn't do a huge amount when I first went home and did have help getting the children to school. I drove again after about a month and that gave me much more freedom. After that, the recovery was quite quick. About six weeks after the operation, everybody came to us for Christmas and I did quite a lot of the cooking. It was only my back which hurt. I still couldn't do things like putting a duvet into the cover but the movement came back in time. "

Some bonuses came from accepting help from family members during the immediate recovery period:

> " The children were eight, seven and nearly three at the time. We are a very close family and my mum and dad came and stayed to help look after the family for the first two weeks. My dad

retrained the children while I was in hospital. He said that I did far too much for them, which was true. He said that they were old enough to tie their laces and taught the youngest one to climb into her car seat because I couldn't lift her for a while. The children wanted to help because they knew I had been poorly. "

For this woman at 67 years old, a mastectomy and immediate autologous latissimus dorsi breast reconstruction was chosen:

" Once the operation was over, I didn't feel too bad. I walked around the next day and went home after a week. I could do most things at home but tired easily. I couldn't reach high things for the first three weeks. I drove again after six weeks. I don't think that the strength in my arm was affected. "

Recovery after a TRAM flap reconstruction can be slower than with other operations:

" I couldn't do a lot when I first went home. My husband did the cooking and looked after me. One of the main things that strikes you is how tired you get. You very quickly find out that you can't do what you thought you could. It is easy to become impatient. I found that I got used to it and settled into making the most of being at home.

I drove again after two months. That wasn't purely because of the physical side. I felt that because I had been out of it for so long, I wasn't sure that I was up to speed mentally.

I went back to work after ten months and had a staggered return. I have been back at work full-time for a year and I do get tired sometimes but I think that I would have done anyway. I have quite a demanding job. There are no practical things that I still find difficult. "

Recovery from any operation can of course be slowed down by complications after surgery. Have a look at pp. 137–145 to find out more about these complications.

All these accounts show that recovery from breast reconstruction can vary enormously, and it's a very individual thing depending on the type of operation you've had and your personal circumstances. Talk as much as possible to the team looking after you and make sure they know about your lifestyle and commitments. Ask them plenty of questions and they'll be able to give you a very good idea about what to expect in the early days after your operation, and in the weeks that lie ahead once you've gone home. Your doctors and nurses are there to help and support you through this time, and to make the experience as easy as possible for you and those close to you.

13 Physiotherapy and rehabilitation after breast reconstruction

- **Movement and exercise will help you to recover more quickly from your surgery.**

- **Your team will explain the kind of exercises you'll need to take to avoid stiffness and to get back to normal.**

- **Your speed of recovery will depend on your own fitness and the type of surgery you've had.**

- **Incorporating your exercises into your daily routine after you've recovered will help to prevent stiffness and maintain full movement.**

With all that is happening to you at the moment and all the decisions you're having to make, physiotherapy may not be at the front of your mind. However, rehabilitation following your surgery is very important, as this woman describes so well:

> " I was given exercises by the physiotherapist in hospital to do at home. I did not realise how important that was. My back became stiff while I was having radiotherapy and I had some more physiotherapy. I wish that I had had more physiotherapy help earlier. "

The aim of the exercises and advice given to you after your operation is to regain normal movement in all areas affected by your operation, and get back to being independent as soon as possible. This is important in restoring some sense of control over what is happening to you. In the early stages in hospital, the whole experience can feel quite overwhelming. Being able to function independently, even in simple things at first, can help towards your recovery. The exercises will be given to you either by a physiotherapist or a breast care nurse.

Every hospital will have their own way of doing things, and the particular exercises and advice you're given after your reconstruction may differ between units. This section contains general advice on your rehabilitation and the importance of physiotherapy, and what you might expect after each type of reconstruction. Always speak to your own surgeon, physiotherapist or breast care nurse about what exercises are appropriate for you to do. If you find that once you've gone home after your operation you're having problems moving your arm, and you haven't had any physiotherapy, ask your breast care nurse about speaking to a physiotherapist. You might be having your reconstruction at the same time as your mastectomy, and know that you're going to have radiotherapy soon after your operation. It's particularly important then to make sure you have good movement in your arm and can get into the position required for your radiotherapy treatment. Speak to your breast care nurse or physiotherapist if in doubt.

Why are exercises important?

In the early stages immediately after your operation you'll probably be given some simple exercises to do to stop your shoulder getting stiff and to help you get back to normal activities. Doing any kind of exercise may be the last thing that you feel like doing. You may be feeing sore and stiff, and you may have wound drains in, which can be uncomfortable. However, even simple things such as brushing your hair with your affected arm may at first seem hard, but will get much easier after doing your exercises.

> 66 The exercises were painful but it became easier. Doing a little bit at a time helps you to get a bit further. 99

You may find that after your operation you tend to protect your affected arm by hugging it in to your body and not using it. Whilst this is a very natural and understandable reaction, it will actually make things worse by causing your shoulder to stiffen up. It can also make the muscles around your upper back and neck become tense and uncomfortable. Gentle exercises started early will help you regain normal posture and enable you to use your arm for light activities, and

170

get your confidence back. It's important that you don't use your arm too much until the wounds have all healed, but it's equally important that you don't let your shoulder stiffen up. Your wounds will probably take about four to six weeks to heal if there aren't any complications.

How soon can I resume my activities after the operation?

You can get back to activities such as reading and knitting as soon as you feel able after your operation. Light housework such as dusting or a little ironing can usually be started after four weeks or so, if you're feeling up to it. Leave heavy housework such as vacuuming and heavy lifting for at least eight weeks. It will always depend on how you're feeling, and check first with your surgeon or physiotherapist if in doubt. Your recovery is exactly that – yours alone, so never compare yourself with anyone else. Expect to be very tired at first, and accept any help that is offered. It can be hard to have to sit back and let your family or friends do your cooking or housework, but if they offer to help, let them, as you'd probably do the same for them!

Both these women had DIEP flaps and found their recovery times quite different:

66 My husband has always been the homemaker but nobody did any more for me than they would normally have done. I was determined to get up and about. I drove after four weeks because I was keen to do so. My family were amazed. 99

66 I found it very difficult to do much at home. This was partly because of the tummy scar which ran from side to side. I found walking hard and getting to the shops at the top of the road after two weeks at home was an achievement. I always had someone with me who could carry the shopping. If I had little goals, it made me do a bit more each time. 99

It's usually possible to start driving after four to six weeks, depending on how you're feeling and what type of reconstruction you had. The main concern is that you're safe and can handle the car in an emergency. Most women find changing gear (if the left arm is affected) and manoeuvres such as reversing and parking the most difficult.

If you have a sedentary job, it may be possible for you to return to work about six to eight weeks after your operation, assuming no other treatment or no complications. If you have an active job, discuss returning to work with your consultant or physiotherapist – it's likely that you'll need to be off work for three to six months or more. This woman took a very sensible approach to returning to work after a DIEP flap:

> 66 I went back to work after six months part-time to begin with and gradually built it up until I did a full day's work. You want to get back to a normal routine and in reality there is no way that you can do this straightaway. It is tiring and I was frightened that people would knock me. 99

Returning to work part-time at first is a good idea, if your work will allow it. In terms of when you'll be able to resume sports and other activities, it does depend on how fit you were before your operation, and whether you have any complications or need other treatments such as chemotherapy or radiotherapy. It will also depend on your own surgeon's views. In general, assuming everything is straightforward, gentle exercise such as walking can be started as soon as you feel able once you go home. Indeed, it can help to get out for a walk and get some fresh air. Sports such as swimming, yoga or pilates can be resumed within two to three months, but you would need to wait at least three months or more before resuming very active sports such as tennis, keep fit, running, and so on. It will depend very much on which type of reconstruction you had and how you're feeling. It will also depend on how much movement you have and which arm is affected. Always check with your surgeon or physiotherapist before resuming any sport.

You might be having your reconstruction at the same time as your mastectomy and then going on to have chemotherapy and/or radiotherapy immediately after your surgery. In this situation, how soon you return to all these activities will depend as much on how your treatment affects you as on how you recover from the surgery itself. It's very important to continue your exercises for quite a long time after your surgery, and especially after radiotherapy. This is because your arm and shoulder can stiffen up for months after your treatment has finished. It's good to have a long-term view, and expect the treatment to take a year out of your life, as this woman who had a DIEP flap describes:

" I had chemotherapy after the operation and it is now a year since the reconstruction. I started going to the gym a few months ago and I do rowing and things like that. The arm on the reconstructed side feels as strong as the other one. "

How long should I do my exercises for?

Keep on doing the exercises once you go home as it may take several weeks until you have normal movement back and you may have some stiffness for several months. If the operation has been straightforward and there have been no complications, there's no reason why you shouldn't regain full movement and get back to normal activities.

" My arm was quite stiff but the movement came back fairly quickly because I did my exercises regularly. "

It's worth incorporating your exercises into your daily life, so that they become a habit and part of your normal routine. Doing them in the shower, or stretching every time you're waiting for the kettle to boil, or when the adverts come on the television, will help to prevent the exercises becoming boring, but will also encourage you to keep exercising and stretching until you regain full movement.

" There comes a terrible boredom threshold [with exercises]. If you don't exercise, you become stiff and you have to realise that you may be in for exercises for the rest of your life. "

Doing some sort of formal exercise that you enjoy will also help, as you can incorporate your specific exercises into more normal routines or sports – swimming, gym work (either using machines on your own or going to exercises classes), pilates, yoga or tai chi, running, and so on.

How can I prepare for my operation?

Your surgeon will make sure you're medically fit for your operation and will discuss the different types of reconstruction and what is available to you from his or her point of view. Try to make sure you have full movement in the affected arm before your surgery. It's worth doing some simple stretching exercises beforehand to improve your movement, especially if you've had previous surgery to your chest or shoulder, or shoulder problems. If you know you have a problem with your shoulder, it's worth mentioning this to your surgeon. It might be possible for you to see a physiotherapist before your operation. This will depend on your hospital. It also helps if you have good general fitness, especially before a longer operation such as the reconstruction using abdominal tissue.

What can I expect after reconstruction with an implant?

Reconstruction using an implant involves placing the implant in a pocket under the muscle on your chest wall (see p. 23). In the days immediately following the operation, it's important to avoid stretching the wound, or using the muscle until the wounds have healed. For the first two to three weeks or so it's generally recommended that you avoid:

- stretching your arm above your head, either forwards or sideways

- stretching your arm behind your back

- lifting or carrying anything heavy with the affected arm

- fastening your bra behind your back – fasten it in front and swivel it round behind you

- pushing or pulling open a heavy door.

If the implant is to be inflated gradually (a tissue expander), this process usually starts about two weeks after your operation. This will depend on your own surgeon. But once the process of inflation has started, you can start using your arm normally, gradually at first and within a pain-free range. It's normal for the front of your chest and your arm to feel tight for several weeks following your operation, but this should improve with exercise and normal use.

Following this type of reconstruction, it's very normal to develop a protective, round-shouldered posture because the front of your chest feels tight and bruised. However, this will generally make you feel even stiffer and can lead to muscle tightness and spasm around your neck and shoulders. As well as doing gentle exercises to keep your arm moving, it helps to be aware of your posture. Try to keep your shoulders relaxed and pulled down. Rolling your shoulders up, back and down regularly will help avoid too much tightness and make you feel less stiff.

What can I expect after reconstruction with a latissimus dorsi flap?

The most important thing to remember after this operation is that the muscle that's been moved to the front of your chest to make your new breast still has its nerve supply, so it's still going to behave like a muscle. It will contract in its new position when you move your arm in certain ways. This can feel very strange indeed! Generally over a period of months, this sensation lessens, although it can remain troublesome for some women.

In its normal position, the muscle acts strongly to bring the arm in to the side of your body and to extend the arm behind your body. The muscle is used in activities that pull your arm in towards the body, such as rowing. It also works strongly to raise your body up such as pushing out of a chair or bath, or climbing. For the first few weeks after the operation it's recommended that you don't stretch or use the muscle that has been taken from your back, or the muscle under your new breast, until they've had a chance to heal. The types of movements and activities to avoid with your affected arm would include:

- stretching above your head or behind your back

- pushing open heavy doors

- pushing yourself off a bed or chair

- carrying anything heavy

- fastening your bra behind your back

- lifting objects onto/off a shelf above your head.

Immediately following the operation, you're most likely to feel discomfort and tightness across your back, sometimes going right down to the small of your back even though the wound is likely to be around your shoulder blade. This is a result of the surgery involved in detaching the muscle from your back so it can be swung round onto your chest wall. A very common description is that it feels like you are

175

wearing a tight corset that you cannot take off. This feeling of tightness is perfectly normal and does wear off, although it can take a few months.

You should get most of the movement back in your arm within six to eight weeks of your operation. It takes much longer for the tight feeling in your back to go away, and indeed, it may feel tighter as the wounds start to heal. Exercises to stretch and move your shoulder blade, combined with deep breathing exercises help to ease the tightness. Once the wounds are healed, try to massage the skin all around the scar on your back and around the side under your armpit. This helps to keep the skin loose and prevent any further tightness.

66 You spend the first year doing exercises, especially with the arm concerned. Massaging the back where the muscle has been taken is also important. 99

The kind of movements that take longest to get back include taking a pullover sweater off over your head, reaching high above your head, pulling shut the car door, stretching forward. However, it's expected that you'll get full movement back in your arm, and be able to resume most if not all of the activities you enjoyed doing before your operation. Activities such as heavy housework, vacuuming and heavy lifting, and sports such as swimming, keep fit, and so on, can be resumed after about three months. This is assuming there are no other complications and your surgeon is happy. And after all your treatment is finished and you're fully recovered, you want to be able to live life to the full and enjoy it, as this woman most certainly does!

66 I can still do very rigorous exercise. I belong to the gym and walk and took up golf after the reconstruction. I explained to the golf pro that I had reconstructive surgery and he understands that I haven't got quite the same follow-through but it's not a problem. The only thing that I stopped deliberately was downhill skiing because I didn't think that I was secure enough to stop myself and also because I have hip arthritis. I don't think that reconstruction has stopped me from doing anything. 99

What can I expect after reconstruction with an abdominal flap (TRAM/DIEP)?

This is major surgery, and there's no point in saying otherwise – described once as like having a hysterectomy and mastectomy at the same time. The initial few days can be really rough, with you feeling sore, stiff, fairly immobile, and wondering about the wisdom of your decision! However, things generally improve quickly once you are up and about, so take the early days one at a time and don't panic.

Your whole abdomen will probably feel very tight and uncomfortable. When you stand or walk this tightness will encourage you to stoop. This is normal, and the tightness will ease. How long it takes for you to be able to stand upright varies between women from a few days to several weeks depending on the extent of the surgery, and your own height and shape. There's no right or wrong, and it's important not to over-stretch your abdominal wound too soon.

> 66 I was fine immediately after the operation. I had to keep still for the first two days, which was hard and stayed in bed for five days altogether. I started walking about after four days and it felt quite strange. I tended to want to shuffle, as opposed to walking properly. 99

Pelvic tilting exercises, where you gently tip your pelvis forwards and backwards whilst keeping your hips bent, can help ease off the tight feeling and any discomfort in your lower back. Once the wound has healed, and usually after at least six weeks, gentle stretching exercises can help ease off any remaining tightness. Try to massage the scar and whole abdomen firmly with moisturising cream. This will help soften the scar and abdominal wall. Avoid any heavy lifting, and any heavy push/pull action, for example vacuuming, for at least six to eight weeks to allow your abdominal muscles to heal.

For the first week or so after your operation it's usually recommended that you avoid stretching your arm above your head so as not to stretch the blood vessels connecting your new breast. Depending on your surgeon, and on how you're doing, you can usually start using your arm normally after the first week or so, gradually at first and within a pain-free range.

<blockquote>
❝ The surgeon was very strict about how much I should do with the arm on the reconstructed side, in case I damaged the blood vessels which had been joined under my arm. ❞
</blockquote>

<blockquote>
❝ You have to be very careful with the affected arm in case you damage the blood vessels. I got out of bed after three or four days and because the arm was weak, it was helpful to have things where I could reach them. I went home after two weeks. ❞
</blockquote>

Carry on doing your exercises once or twice a day for as long as you feel the benefit of them, and certainly until you regain full movement. It is expected that unless you had any restrictions before your operation, you should regain full movement in your arm within a few weeks. Returning to full activities will take much longer, six months or more. However, if you have any complications with your wounds it may take longer – again there's no right or wrong. It's very important to note that everyone reacts differently to this operation. Some examples of this may be found on p. 166.

How far you want to take your exercises after your operation is up to yourself and will depend on your own lifestyle. If you're keen to do more strengthening exercises for your abdominal muscles, speak to your physiotherapist, or a fitness instructor if you go to a gym. Pilates exercises are excellent for developing strength in the deep, protective abdominal muscles, and encouraging good posture.

What can I expect after reconstruction with an SGAP flap?

This is a much less common type of reconstruction (see p. 96). In terms of using your arm, the same advice applies as after an abdominal reconstruction. The most important thing is to avoid over-stretching your arm in the early days so as to not to pull on the blood vessels connecting your new breast. The wound on your buttock will make sitting down and bending your hip uncomfortable at first. Try to avoid bending your hip forwards too much until your wounds have healed. This can take four to six weeks. Once the wounds have healed, massaging them with moisturising cream will keep them soft and supple. In the long term, because there are no major functional implications of losing the muscle from your buttock, you should be able to get back to all normal activities after three months or so.

> " I am fit and supple from doing yoga but found not being able to do things like lift my arm far quite frustrating. Things like shopping on my own were difficult at first. Using a trolley or a suitcase on wheels was helpful. You need to be prepared for several months of recovery and do have to take it easy. The recovery was slow, but not desperately so. "

What further information might be useful?

You should be able to get all the information you need about exercises and rehabilitation, both in the short- and long-term, from your physiotherapist. If you don't have direct access to a physiotherapist, you should be able to access physiotherapy services through your breast care nurse, consultant or GP. Another resource that you may find useful, especially as you can use it in your own home, is an exercise video/DVD designed especially for women who have had breast reconstruction, called Fighting Breast Cancer – We Can Help. Details of this are on p. 220.

14 Anxieties and concerns about breast reconstruction

- The diagnosis and treatment of breast cancer is a very distressing and emotional experience for most women.

- Breast reconstruction is not a remedy for all your worries and concerns about recovering from your cancer.

- Many women find that breast reconstruction is a very positive experience.

- You may find it difficult to make a decision about breast reconstruction.

- Your breast team will be able to help you make your decision.

- It's better not to go ahead with immediate reconstruction if you can't make up your mind.

In this section we'll take a look at some of the psychological issues that face women who are thinking about breast reconstruction and, in many cases, their partners too. We'll consider the worries, anxieties and concerns that many women report throughout the process of reconstruction, especially during the period of decision-making and later when adjusting to their reconstructed breast. It's important to remember that deciding to undergo reconstructive surgery is a very personal and individual experience and you might find that not all of these issues apply to you. You may also have some worries that aren't touched upon here. If this should be the case, your breast care team and the organisations listed on pp. 215–217 can offer advice and support.

The psychological impact of mastectomy

It's well known that the diagnosis and treatment of breast cancer can be a very distressing and emotional experience. Throughout this time, and beyond, you're likely to experience a wide range of emotions. Some of these may be positive (such as relief following a good treatment outcome and feelings towards friends and family offering their practical and emotional support), whilst others, such as fear, anxiety, sadness, uncertainty, frustration, indecision, anger and helplessness can be much more difficult to handle.

As well as concerns about their diagnosis, many women worry about the impact that treatment can have upon their appearance and the way they feel about their body. Undergoing a mastectomy can be especially difficult, and some women report this as being the most distressing and emotional aspect of their cancer journey. Research suggests that about one in three women who undergo mastectomy experience significant levels of psychological distress at some stage. In a society that seems to place so much emphasis upon appearance, reactions to a mastectomy can be very complex. Some women adjust very well, whilst others find this much harder. For some women, their breasts are integral to their feelings of femininity, attractiveness and sexuality. They might also be associated with breastfeeding and rearing children. Other women place less importance on these aspects, but still fear that loss of a breast or both breasts can feel like an assault on their body image – the internal view they have of their body. They worry that losing a breast will leave them feeling unbalanced and incomplete, as well as acting as a reminder of their cancer and its treatment.

Many women find that an external breast prosthesis is a good solution to their concerns, but others worry about using a prosthesis – concerned that other people will notice it, that it might fall out or that it might restrict their choice of clothing and activities. And a prosthesis may be a reminder of the surgery. Breast reconstruction offers the chance to recreate a breast shape and often provides psychological benefits in terms of improved quality of life and body image for those women who want to avoid an external prosthesis. But this isn't always the case, and reconstruction isn't necessarily a solution for all of the challenges associated with mastectomy. Undergoing breast reconstruction is a major commitment, and both the physical and psychological outcomes of surgery are hard to predict. This can sometimes make it very difficult for you to decide whether or not to undergo reconstructive surgery.

Making decisions about breast reconstruction

For some women, the decision whether or not to undergo breast reconstruction can feel like the first genuine choice they've had since hearing their diagnosis. But this isn't a decision any woman wants to be confronted with. Nobody wants to be diagnosed with breast cancer, and consenting to undergo a mastectomy might not feel like a genuine choice.

You may face a number of difficulties when making a decision about reconstruction because:

- The decision has the potential to influence the way you will look for the rest of your life.

- The options are likely to be presented soon after the diagnosis of cancer has been given and various treatment choices are being discussed. Even if it's anticipated, hearing the diagnosis is still likely to come as a shock. This is a natural reaction to bad news.

- Many women report feeling as if the doctors were talking about somebody else – a sense that 'this isn't really happening to me'.

- The range of options about the types of procedures and the timing of surgery can sometimes make decision-making both complex and daunting. Making the choice is likely to involve having to consider complicated information and to weigh up numerous alternatives. It can be hard to take in – and remember – all the information that is being provided.

- Even women who are usually very decisive and find it easy to make complicated or major decisions can find themselves overwhelmed by the choices available to them at this time.

- Some women worry about making the wrong choice and this can add to the anxieties already being experienced at this emotional time.

There are several ways that women who are finding it particularly difficult to make their decision can find help. These include information-seeking, preparation and talking to other people (see also p. 203).

Information preferences

People vary in the amount of information they need to be able to make a decision. Some people want as much information as possible and can find it worrying and frustrating not to have this to hand. Others want much less detail and find that too much information can be cause anxiety. It can be useful to think carefully about the type and level of information that you want before making your choice. Research has shown that having sufficient, appropriate information can help patients to have a feeling of control about their cancer and its treatment. It's also thought that those women who are more satisfied with the information they had about reconstruction and felt they had sufficient time to make their decision are more likely to be satisfied that they've made the right choice.

Preparing for discussions about surgery

Discussing major, personal issues with healthcare professionals such as surgeons can feel difficult and cause anxiety, so it's useful to prepare yourself in advance for any consultations. It can be very helpful to draw up a list of questions you want to ask. This can be particularly helpful when the consultation involves discussions about reconstructive surgery (see p. 204).

Making a 'good' decision

Remember that when you are making your decision, you're trying to make the choice that's best for you, not one that is best for anyone else. One way of looking at a decision is to think of a good decision as one that you won't regret later.

The things that are important to you

Think about the things that are really important to you. These might include the views of family and friends, activities such as sports, your work or the types of clothing you like to wear. Thinking about the impact that undergoing breast reconstruction (or not) might have upon these things might help to clarify your choice.

The advantages and disadvantages as you see them

It can also be useful to draw up a list of what you, personally, see as the advantages and disadvantages of having breast reconstruction, followed by the pros and cons of each type of procedure. This is your personal list – there aren't any right and wrong answers since what is an advantage to one person might be a disadvantage to another. It's important to write the list down, rather than just think about it, because the process of putting pen to paper will help you to clarify your thoughts.

How would you react to possible scenarios?

It can be helpful to take time to try to think about how you might feel or react to a number of possible scenarios, for example:

- How might you feel if you needed to have more surgery than you had anticipated?

- What would you do if the results of surgery weren't quite as you had hoped?

This can be difficult, and while thinking about things is not the same as experiencing them directly, it can help to clarify your choice and possibly prepare you if they should actually happen. It's also helpful to talk these through with other people, for example your partner or breast care nurse.

What should you do if you are still unsure?

Throughout your decision-making it's worth remembering that the option of breast reconstruction will still be available to you in the future. If you're unsure whether to go ahead with the surgery, you might prefer to put the decision 'on hold' for the time being. Circumstances might change, you might find that you can clarify your preferences more easily in the future, and the decision might be much clearer and easier to make at a later date. Delaying the decision at this stage can be an effective way of coping with some of the stress around your diagnosis and could be preferable to making a rushed decision that might be regretted later.

Having made your decision, you might still think of questions and concerns – before or after surgery has taken place – and you should still ask your breast care team about these. If you've decided to undergo delayed reconstruction, you may have to wait a matter of weeks or months before the surgery takes place. It can be helpful to meet with your surgeon once more before the surgery is due to take place, as an opportunity to raise any further questions you may have.

The experience of breast reconstruction

Having realistic expectations

A reconstructed breast is not the same as your natural breast, and it's not a true replacement. Women who've undergone reconstruction can still experience a sense of loss for their breast. Those who expect that a reconstructed breast will look and feel the same as the breast they've lost are likely to be disappointed. Having realistic expectations of the outcome of surgery is vital. To this end, it is useful to discuss your expectations with your surgical team since they'll be able to determine whether your hopes are likely to be met. They'll be able to correct any of your misunderstandings, and it will help them to have a better understanding of what you hope the surgery will achieve.

One of the difficulties surrounding breast reconstruction is that it's very difficult to describe how a reconstructed breast will actually feel. Photographs can give you a clear idea of what it might look like, but it's hard to describe and understand physical sensations until you've experienced them. Some women describe experiencing a tingling sensation in their reconstructed breast for some time after the initial surgery. For others this is more painful, and some women have no sensations at all. Talking to women who have undergone surgery can give you an indication, but there's no guarantee that your own experiences will be the same as theirs.

Coping with your emotions

Any type of surgery typically provokes anxiety and it's natural to feel nervous before the operation takes place. Anxiety is particularly great amongst women undergoing breast reconstruction because of the high hopes about the outcome of the surgery. It's not unusual to feel tearful around the time of surgery, both before and after it's taken place, and it might sometimes feel as if you are on a rollercoaster of emotions. There are likely to be days when you feel down, and others when you feel very well and maybe elated at the results of surgery. In the following account, a woman describes how she felt during this time and offers some useful advice:

> " You need to take it one day at a time and be allowed to have moments when you are upset. Crying is not being weak. You have to be allowed to be like that in order to build yourself up again. You need time to get back to normal and not think you are different to everybody else. There will be knock backs. "

Seeing your reconstructed breast for the first time

Looking at the results of surgery for the first time can be a significant event and a time of mixed emotions – typically relief that the surgery is over, that the disease has been removed and that a breast shape remains. Women undergoing a delayed reconstruction are often delighted that the distress caused by the mastectomy has been alleviated. It can be a good idea to look at the results of the surgery for the first time whilst still in the hospital environment. Massaging cream into the scars can be a way of getting used to touching the reconstructed area while also helping to keep the scars soft. It's important to remember that the initial outcome of surgery may not be the same as final results since scars take time to settle and further procedures may be needed.

Getting used to your new breast

Even if the results of your surgery are better than expected, it can take some time to adjust to the look and feel of a reconstructed breast. Some women soon feel very comfortable with it and incorporate it into their body image well. Others find this harder, and the process of adjustment can be a prolonged and enduring one, sometimes taking a year or more depending on the amount of surgery. Again, it can be helpful to talk to your breast care team if you're having problems getting used to your new breast. They may be able to help you with your concerns themselves, or can direct you towards other sources of support when needed.

There are many different ways of coping with the worries and concerns associated with breast reconstruction. What helps one woman will not necessarily be helpful for another and similarly, what's helpful for an individual woman might change over time.

Keeping a record of your experiences

Some women find it helpful to keep a diary throughout this period as a way of recording and reflecting on their experiences and feelings.

Others find it helpful to keep a photographic record or journal. This might sound a little strange, since we usually take photographs of happy occasions such as weddings and birthdays, rather than difficult and sometimes distressing experiences such as this. This woman found this to be very therapeutic:

> " When we came home, as soon as the dressings were taken off, I decided that I wanted to keep a photo diary because I wanted to be able to see the progress. If I had a down day, I wanted to be able to look back and see the improvements. It was very helpful because there are times when you don't think you are improving and its good to look back and compare it with other times. I kept the photo diary until the uplift operation had been done on the other side and the whole thing was almost complete. It would probably even be helpful to compare again because another six months have passed. I have found that things change constantly. None of it stays static. For me, it gives me confidence to look back. If you do look at yourself in the mirror, you do not look perfect but I was never perfect. It helped me; other people may feel differently about it. It does help if you feel comfortable about looking at yourself objectively. "

Other people

Decisions about cancer treatment, including those about breast reconstruction, don't take place in isolation. It's likely that other people, especially partners, family and friends, have been distressed by the news of the cancer diagnosis. They might also have their own views about breast reconstruction that could influence your own decision. Although this is your own choice, you might want to ask those people who are important to you, such as your husband or partner, what they think about it. It's usually far better to ask them and discuss it with them than to assume you know what they think.

Sometimes women worry about being a burden on other people during the post-operative period, when they aren't able to carry out their usual routine. Family and friends often report that they want to provide practical support, for example helping with shopping, driving and caring for children, since this helps them to feel involved and to demonstrate their support. This is illustrated by the husband of a woman who underwent reconstructive surgery:

> " The husband's role is a supporting role. You can't really help with the decision-making. It has to be the wife's decision. There is not a lot you can do about the frustrating times, other than trying to be there and being supportive. "

What about the children's reactions?

Women often worry about their children during this time, in particular whether to tell them about the surgery and how they will react. This woman who had reconstructive surgery describes her experiences in relation to her young children:

> " My daughter, aged 5, wouldn't talk to me about the operation. It did upset her and she didn't like it when I had to go into hospital again. My three year old son would ask me point blank how things were. I think the fact that the children expected life to carry on helped me to carry on. I had to keep it together for them. The children were wonderful and have seen the reconstruction at every stage …. They just take it for granted that is what you look like and you are Mum. "

Handling other people's reactions

Dealing with other people's reactions to the surgery can be a significant event when they see the results for the first time. Some people who know about the surgery might be intrigued, ask questions or hope to see the results for themselves. It's worth thinking about how you might handle such situations in advance. A polite, prepared response and a deliberate change in the topic of conversation can let others know if you would prefer not to discuss it in detail, if that's the case.

Intimate relationships

Partners of women who've undergone breast reconstruction have reported the concerns and feelings of isolation that they experience during the process. Although they want to support their partner while she makes her decision and undergoes surgery, they might also want to talk to somebody about how they are feeling themselves, but worry about over-burdening their partner at this time. Often they don't know anyone else who has had breast reconstruction and might feel uncomfortable about talking about the surgery to their friends.

They might also feel worried about hurting their partner or opening scars if they touch the reconstructed breast. The woman herself might also be worrying about intimate relationships after surgery. She might be feeling conscious of the reconstructed breast and worrying about possible pain and levels of sensation. In this situation she may interpret her partner's behaviour as a rejection or of evidence that he no longer finds her attractive. This misunderstanding can lead to communication problems and heightened anxiety for both partners. Although it might be difficult, creating an atmosphere of open and honest communication between partners throughout the whole process can make things easier in the longer term and offers the potential for both to benefit from the support of the other partner.

This woman who had reconstructive surgery describes how both she and her husband took some time to get used to her reconstructed breast:

> 66 My husband has never been into great physical beauty, he is not that sort of person. I was never concerned that he might look at me and think 'how revolting'. He will ask me why I am spending time doing my hair because it doesn't matter. I had the reconstruction because I still wanted to look sexy. I didn't want to have something on my chest that I was ashamed of because it was hideous. The reconstruction has not affected our sex life. It doesn't feel the same, but I have got used to the difference. It did take a bit of time. My husband used to avoid it a bit and I had to tell him that he didn't have to. It does feel different – like someone touching you through several layers. The breast can feel a bit cold because it doesn't warm up. I do notice it in summer when it is hot and I have a cool breast. 99

Women who aren't in an intimate relationship can face the dilemma of whether (and when) to tell a new partner that they've had a mastectomy and reconstructive surgery. This can be very worrying and, as ever, there are no right or wrong answers. Talking about intimacy and sexual issues can be difficult in any circumstances, but a diagnosis of cancer can sometimes compound this, and worrying about a partner's reaction to breast reconstruction can make this even harder.

Professional support

Specialist nurses are trained to offer emotional support to all women facing breast reconstruction. In addition, some women can benefit from referral onwards for further psychological support – for example, those finding it very difficult to decide whether or not to have the surgery, experiencing difficulty in adjusting to their appearance or needing help with a relationship after surgery. Your breast care team will be able to help you with these referrals.

Members of your breast care team or your GP might be able to help you with any worries or concerns you have about intimacy or sexual issues, but again it can be difficult to talk to healthcare professionals about this personal subject. In these circumstances, the organisations listed on pp. 215–217 will be able to help.

Conclusion

For many women who've faced a diagnosis of breast cancer, reconstructive surgery is a very positive experience, and one that can help to reduce their distress. But it must be remembered that this is a major surgical procedure and it's not necessarily a remedy for all of the anguish caused by the diagnosis and mastectomy. Taking time to make an informed decision can reap benefits in terms of improved adjustment to the reconstructed breast after surgery. Making the decision is sometimes difficult and your breast care team are there to help you. They can provide information, arrange meetings with other women who've been through the same experience and make referrals to other sources of support. It's important for women, their partners and families, and healthcare professionals to remember that breast reconstruction is a major commitment and it's quite normal for women to feel anxious or concerned about it.

15 Mastectomy without reconstruction

- **Many women don't have reconstruction after mastectomy because they feel it's not important to them.**

- **Your breast care nurse will be able to provide practical advice to help you feel more confident after your operation.**

- **You may find it helpful to get first hand information from other women who have recovered from mastectomy.**

- **You can get lots of information about bras, prostheses, clothing, exercises and your recovery from your breast care nurse.**

If you're unable to have breast reconstruction or would prefer not to have it, it is possible to live successfully with a mastectomy. In this section we'll discuss this option and give you tips from people who have done this.

Making the decision

66 I was 50 when I chose to have a mastectomy, rather than a lumpectomy and radiotherapy. I did not know anyone who had had breast cancer before, so had no pre-conceived ideas. My decision was made partly because I did not want to have radiotherapy but also because I thought that I didn't have the need for the breast any more. I just wanted to get rid of it and get on with life. Breast reconstruction was mentioned to me but I

was quite happy not to have it. The loss of a breast did not concern me. I am a country person, not a fashion person, so not having a cleavage didn't worry me. My husband was very happy to go along with this decision.

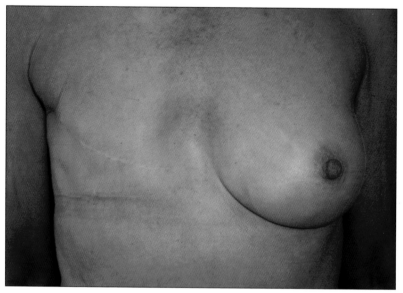

A right mastectomy scar

For this woman, the suggestion of an operation on the unaffected breast to match the reconstructed breast influenced the decision:

I was only just coming to terms with the news that I needed a mastectomy when I was given a load of information about breast reconstruction as well. As I had never thought about this before, I didn't have any idea about which I should have. I hadn't realised that they would have to take tissue from another part of the body to rebuild the missing breast.

With someone small-breasted like me, they would probably want to operate on my good breast as well to match the reconstructed breast. The fact that you can make someone perfect and whole again is not necessarily true. It was a decision that I wanted to go and think about. My top priority was not to get breast cancer

again. The physical issue for me was that I didn't really want to have the other breast operated on. I was 49 and had a very good partner. I now know that after a mastectomy you do get scar tissue, some discomfort and a lack of feeling and I didn't want my other breast to feel odd as well.
"

Your feelings about your appearance

We all feel differently about our bodies and what they could look like after an operation. This can be a very important issue for some and unimportant to others although there's no right way to feel (see p. 180).

"	Your own feelings about body image are important. I am lucky enough to be quite confident about my body image. Having a big bust is not going to change my life. I have had a very good life and my partner is happy. I know that people have partners for whom this is very important and then it would have to be taken into account.
"

"	I wasn't too worried about the appearance of a mastectomy because I have always been fairly flat-chested and worn padded bras. My husband wouldn't have married me if he had wanted someone with big breasts. The fact that I had seen my colleague coping with a prosthesis also helped me to decide. I was told that I could always have a reconstruction later if I wanted one.
"

Making the mastectomy more acceptable

There are several practical ways to make having a mastectomy more acceptable and to help you feel more confident with your new appearance. These include:

- having a suitable, well fitted and pretty bra
- having a well fitted prosthesis
- making adjustments to your clothes if necessary.

Before your operation

Talking to your breast care nurse

Do take time to talk over the practical aspects of your operation with your breast care nurse. She'll be able to give you a realistic idea about what to expect in terms of what sort of scarring you'll have, length of time in hospital and how long you'll need to recover afterwards, depending on your lifestyle. She should also be able to show you photographs of someone who's had a mastectomy, advise you about suitable bras and show you a prosthesis if you'd like to see one. She'll also listen to and help you explore any concerns you have. If possible, take someone close to you with you for these appointments. Two heads are often better than one.

Talking to another patient

Another very helpful way to get used to the idea of a mastectomy and gain more first-hand information, support and tips, can be to ask your breast care nurse to introduce you to someone else who's already had this operation. Someone who has been through this already will understand how you may be feeling and can help talk through your concerns as well as tell you how they coped and show you that it's possible to recover well afterwards. No two experiences will be exactly the same, but this can still be a useful thing to do.

> " I am the fifth teacher in my school to have been diagnosed with breast cancer in the past four years. We have all had different treatments and when I was told that I needed a mastectomy, I knew about my colleagues' experiences. You never think that it will happen to you. I was told that I could have a breast reconstruction if I wanted. The fact that I had seen my colleague coping with a prosthesis also helped me. "

It is also fine not to wish to talk to others:

> " I did not meet anyone who had a mastectomy before the operation because I didn't want anyone else's experiences. I could then cope with it my way. "

Breast prostheses

What is a prosthesis?

A prosthesis is a synthetic breast form that will fit into your bra cup to replace either the whole breast or part of it. They're mostly made from silicone gel, which has an outer film cover, and come in different weights, sizes, shapes and skin tones. Self-adhesive prostheses are also available.

Everyone should be offered a prosthesis after a mastectomy, and it's your personal choice whether you decide to wear one. Initially, while the scar is healing, you'll be offered a 'comfy' or 'softie'. This is a lightweight prosthesis that fills out your bra but it's not heavy. Because of the lightness, it might move upwards in your bra cup but you can either pin or sew it into you bra cup to hold it more securely. These are usually worn for about six to eight weeks until the scar is comfortable and well healed.

Your breast care nurse should advise you when you're fully healed and ready to be fitted with the silicone prosthesis. These are either fitted by your breast care nurses or by an appliance fitter in the hospital. These are free of charge to NHS patients.

Getting a suitable bra

One of things that will help you cope with a mastectomy is wearing a bra that holds the prosthesis properly and feels comfortable. It helps you forget that you're wearing a prosthesis by making your chest look symmetrical when dressed.

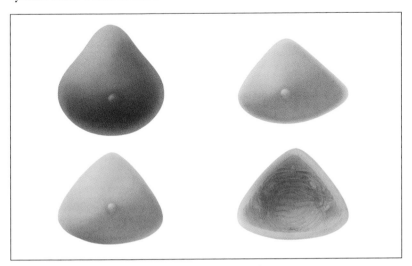

Examples of commercially available breast prostheses

Buying from the high street shops

It's quite possible to wear bras and swimwear bought from high street shops, if you know what you need. Here are some important features to look for:

- a full cup, which will cover the prosthesis
- a firm or elasticated top edge to the cup to hold the prosthesis
- make sure that the side of the bra under your arm is deep enough
- an underband that is at least 1 cm deep
- at least two hooks to fasten the bra, with more for larger sizes
- straps that are not too thin
- a bra that separates your breasts between the cups.

If your bra already fits this description, then it may not be necessary to get a new one. The best way to check is to show one to your breast care nurse when discussing the operation.

You should always ask an assistant to measure you before buying any bras. Assistants in department store lingerie departments or specialist underwear shops have often been trained to measure for bras after mastectomy and will understand any concerns you may have. Ask your breast care nurse to recommend your best local shops for this, and the best timing for being fitted with your bras.

Using and buying specially designed mastectomy bras and swimwear

Some women prefer to buy specially designed mastectomy bras, swimwear and accessories, which have all the features mentioned earlier. These can be bought either from mail-order companies or personally by visiting their shops. The advantage of specially designed garments is that they already have pockets sewn into the bra cup that hold the prosthesis securely.

Fitting pockets into bras

If your chosen bras are unpocketed and you want to sew your own pockets into your bras, then choose a stretchable material to sew across the back of the cup. Make sure that the bra cup is not pulled too tightly across the back. This could distort the shape of your bra and spoil your appearance. You can then insert the prosthesis into the cup from the side. Another way to hold a prosthesis in your bra cup is to sew two ribbons, crossed across the back of your bra cup – again, not too tightly.

Some hospitals will sew pockets into your bras for you. It is worth asking whether this service is available and how many pockets they are prepared to do.

Some people switch between mastectomy bras and swimwear and high street bras, depending on what they are doing.

> 66 I wear mastectomy bras with pockets. This year, for the first time, I feel quite confident and do not really think about it any more. When I go running, I wear a loose T-shirt and a sports bra without a prosthesis. Prostheses get a bit hot and sweaty when you run. I don't swim a huge amount but, after talking to a friend who also had a mastectomy, I don't wear a prosthesis. Because I am small, if I wear a swimming costume with an insert bra which is quite stiff, I can get away with nothing inside it. My fear is that I don't want to embarrass anyone else. 99

> 66 To begin with, I bought a sports bra because my colleague had told me that it was as good as any to wear with a comfy. When I was ready for my proper prosthesis, I bought mastectomy bras and a mastectomy swimming costume. I have bras which are white, black and flesh-coloured, depending on the occasion. The prosthesis is fine. Sometimes I forget that I have got it on because it is so comfortable. I wear contact lenses and taking all the prosthesis paraphernalia on holiday is just another extension of that. I do change in communal changing rooms. The scar is more of a problem when I have no clothes on. I tend not to look. My husband says that he is not concerned about it. 99

> 66 I bought mastectomy bras through mail order and had no problem wearing the comfy initially. It looked very similar to the other breast. I felt pleased when I first put the heavy prosthesis on because I felt normal again. I have pockets in my bra and have no problems with any activity, including riding. Communal changing rooms do not concern me at all. To my mind, that is somebody else's problem. I wear a mastectomy swimming costume, which is fine. 99

The early days after your surgery

One of the most daunting things to face is looking at your new appearance and coping with your reaction to it. It's often helpful to do this for the first time while you're still in hospital. That way, if you want to, you may be able to have the help and support of either the breast care nurse or one of the nurses on the ward.

" I remember, in the days leading up to the mastectomy, treasuring my left breast a little bit. I thought that I should make the most of it because it was going.

I had to be brave to look in the mirror for the first time after the operation, but I made myself do that quite early on. I tried to feel interested in the operation scientifically to distract myself from self-pity. I thought that it was amazing that they had stitched me up like that and thought that it was OK. I showed my husband straight away and we got over that hurdle.

Over the subsequent three years, I still catch myself in the mirror and am quite surprised. I am not sure that you really get used to it. If I walk down the street, I see people with a lot worse wrong that is obvious, so I can't really complain about it. "

Coming home from hospital

The amount of time that you may spend in hospital after a mastectomy can vary. Women now often go home with drainage tubes still in the wound. The drains are put in during the operation to keep the wound dry and help healing. If necessary, they can be taken out at home. Do remember that you are likely to feel tired and weak at first.

" I went home the day after the operation with a drain in and it does take a while to recover physically. We went on holiday in France after a couple of weeks and I spent that time recuperating. I was going through the psychological aspects of it and it was lovely to have the family to support me. Having children to distract me was probably the key to getting back to normal. "

" I went home five days after the operation with the drain still in. Once the drain was removed, I did have some serous fluid collecting under the scar but after having it drained once, it dried up. I could do quite a lot when I got home. "

" I wasn't in a lot of pain after the operation, although the drain was a bit sore. I went home after two days with a drain in and it was a relief when that was taken out. I felt a bit wobbly when I first got home. "

Fluid drainage

Once your drainage tubes have been removed, it is not unusual for fluid to collect under the scar. This can be drawn off easily and often painlessly, if necessary, as an outpatient.

Your exercises

You should be given advice before leaving hospital about the use of your arm and what exercises will help your recovery (see p. 169). It's important to try to do these regularly. The fact that you have not had a breast reconstruction does not mean that the exercises are any less important, and it's helpful to carry on doing them long after the wound has healed and you've finished all your treatment.

" I did the exercises that I was taught regularly but I wasn't prepared for the fact that my arm became painful and the scar tightened up over the next few days as the tendons tightened. It did improve with some physiotherapy. "

" My arm was easy to move at the beginning but as the tissue healed, it tightened up and I had to do the exercises. Sometimes you wonder whether it will ever move properly. The numbness around the scar and back doesn't actually go. It can just feel odd and uncomfortable. "

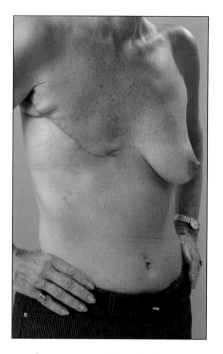

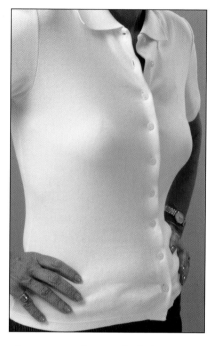

Appearance undressed after a mastectomy

Appearance of a prosthesis in a correctly fitting bra and clothes

Resuming your activities and returning to work

There is no right amount of time to take before resuming previous activities and returning to work. This depends on wound healing, how you feel and what advice you have been given. Going back to work and facing colleagues can be both daunting and very tiring.

66 I went back to work after five months and worked part-time for the first two months. At first I felt as though I wasn't up to speed with the work. It is a year since the operation and I am happy and comfortable with it. It is part of how things are and that is it. I have achieved my aim of going back to work and getting on with life. I do have times when I feel down about it but would not want reconstruction now because I would rather avoid operations if possible. 99

200

> My work involves looking after horses and I went back to riding after five weeks. I felt as though I had freedom again. It is now three years since the surgery and I can do everything.

Making some adjustments to the type of clothes you choose can help your confidence initially:

> I work in a university and have to give presentations. I remember giving the first one after going back to work and being very aware of myself. I was standing up in front of a group of people when I was just getting used to wearing a prosthesis and wondered whether it looked right. I was not worried if somebody asked me about the mastectomy but did not want to draw attention to myself. I bought a lot of jackets in the first year because I was always worrying about whether the prosthesis would slip down or somebody would notice if there was a problem. The jackets helped my confidence and as I got more comfortable, I changed the type of prosthesis. It takes time to get used to it and find what is right.

Here are some final thoughts about having a mastectomy:

> I think that it is very important to be very open and talk about the mastectomy. I talked with my husband a lot. I did joke with very close friends and a sense of humour helps. It is good to take each day as it comes, be positive and do the exercises. It is important to get on with it because you have been given another chance.

> Having got myself so that I am comfortable, I don't particularly want the body change that a reconstruction would bring. I am also scared of playing about with what I have got. I have got one breast that is fine and I would not want to end up looking at it and thinking that actually I prefer what I had before.

Some good things have come out of having a mastectomy. It has made me very aware and empathetic. The really nice thing that I have learned is that I thought when you have something bad happen to you, you would probably never feel like a nice young carefree person again. You can come out of it and begin to feel your old bubbly self again. It takes time, but as long as you let yourself go with the flow, things improve. Don't expect too much too soon.

"

16 Getting all your information together quickly

- Don't be pushed into making a decision about breast reconstruction, as it has to be the right decision for you.

- It's important to make a checklist of questions and to take someone with you to listen when you meet your surgeon.

- If the reconstruction you want can't be carried out in your local Breast Unit, you can ask to be referred to another unit.

- Many women find it very helpful to talk to others who have had breast reconstruction carried out, and to see the results for themselves.

- Photographs and written material can help you understand more about breast reconstruction.

You've just been given a new diagnosis and you're facing decisions about different treatments at a very stressful time, or you may be someone who's considering breast reconstruction some time after your mastectomy, at your leisure. Whichever situation you find yourself in, it's vital to remember that to make the right decision for you, you need to have realistic expectations of what breast reconstruction involves and what results to expect, including possible complications.

It's vitally important to have plenty of time to weigh up your options and what they would mean for you before coming to a decision. It's often really helpful to take a friend or relative with you to listen to the discussions and to support you in your decision-making. Likewise, writing down your questions and the answers can help you when recalling the discussion afterwards.

Here are some patients' thoughts:

" I was only given one option but probably could have had a choice of different reconstructions if I had asked more questions. In an ideal world, people should have the chance to consider all the options, as well as seeing people who have had them by the same surgeon. With hindsight, I did not have enough information to make a balanced judgement. The issues that I did not know about were how much additional surgery I would have and how long the whole process took. People need to have realistic expectations and understand that the reconstructed breast may be a good imitation but not exactly the same. What is good for one person may not be good for another. "

" I had two weeks to make up my mind, although I could have had longer. I didn't want to keep putting off the inevitable. It is hard, because you try to cope with the diagnosis of cancer and all the worries that brings, and at the same time try to decide between two different procedures. It is impossible to know what the outcome is going to be. It was never an option for me not to have the reconstruction. I knew that even though it was hard, in a way it was probably quite good for me because it made me focus on something other than the cancer. This was something that I could control and decide. I thought up loads of questions and took my sister with me to the appointments when we were discussing the options. "

When getting your information together, here's a checklist of helpful questions to ask:

- Is breast reconstruction suitable for me?
- What are my options, and why?
- Can this be done immediately or should I wait until later?
- What would these operations involve?
- How long will I be in hospital?

- How will it affect my recovery?

- How long will I be off work?

- How long will all this take?

- Will breast reconstruction affect my lifestyle?

- What are the possible risks and complications of breast reconstruction, compared with the benefits?

- Can I see pictures of the different types of reconstruction?

- Can I speak to patients who have had breast reconstruction already?

- Will breast reconstruction delay other treatments?

- What experience do your surgeons have of breast reconstruction?

- Are there any other options you don't provide here?

Here are some different avenues to explore:

Your breast clinic

If you've already been referred to your breast clinic and no one's mentioned breast reconstruction, ask your surgeon whether it's suitable for you and whether it's done at your hospital. There's a big variation in the amount carried out across the country and your chances of being offered breast reconstruction depend on resources available locally. Some surgeons are trained to do both breast cancer surgery and breast reconstruction (oncoplastic surgeons). In other centres the breast surgeon will do the breast surgery and their colleagues in plastic surgery will do the breast reconstruction, either at the same time or at a later date. Because there's quite a range of different types of breast reconstruction, it is possible that your hospital won't be able to offer you a full choice of operations. If you're interested in finding out more about one particular type of breast reconstruction which isn't available at your hospital, you should ask where it is performed. Your surgeon can refer you there to find out more about it. If breast reconstruction isn't available locally at all, you can ask to be referred to the nearest centre for your treatment. If you are unsure about the options you have been given, don't forget that you can always ask to be referred to another centre for a second opinion.

> In talking this through with my surgeon, I was told about his colleague who was an oncoplastic surgeon and could do the two operations of a mastectomy and breast reconstruction at the same time. I asked to go and see this surgeon and he was happy to refer me. The second surgeon suggested that I should have a lumpectomy first, as I had not had radiotherapy in the past and he also went through all the different types of reconstruction. He agreed with me that because of my large droopy breasts, the DIEP flap would give me a more realistic reconstruction. He said that if I did want to have that, he would refer me to a plastic surgeon who specialised in it.

Your breast care nurse

Breast care nurses should be available in the Breast Unit. They are able to give you the time to discuss your options more fully, look at photographs of different breast reconstructions and talk about all the practical aspects of the procedures and your recovery, as well as providing you with emotional support. These appointments are often separate from your consultation with the surgeon and this gives you a good opportunity to think about any questions which you may not have asked already. You'll have a chance to run through them in more detail with your nurse in a more relaxed, informal environment. If you're not introduced to the breast care nurse in the clinic, ask how you can arrange to meet later. They should also be able to provide you with written material and sometimes videos to help with your decision-making.

Talking to other patients

As well as talking to members of the Breast Unit and looking at photographs, some women find it very helpful to talk to patients who have already been through breast reconstruction, to ask about their experiences and recovery at first hand. Contact with these patients can be made in a number of ways: through your breast care nurse, through patient support groups or through a number of national organisations that can put you in touch with a range of women. If you're considering more than one type of breast reconstruction, it can be helpful to meet several patients to compare their experiences and to have an opportunity to look at the results of their different procedures. Support groups also often have books and leaflets about breast reconstruction that you can have or borrow.

" I was offered the opportunity to talk to other patients who had undergone breast reconstruction, and seized that opportunity. The surgeon told me to go and have a chat with them, have a look at their reconstructions and then make my mind up. He said that it was a big decision and I should take my time. I was told that there were two options and spoke to one person for each type. As soon as I phoned the first person up, she was brilliant. She was positive, reassuring and full of energy. I went to see her and we chatted as if we were old friends. I knew when I saw her breast that I did not want to have that type of reconstruction. Seeing this in the flesh as well as in the photographs was very helpful. I then spoke to the lady who had a latissimus dorsi breast reconstruction three years earlier. She was full of energy and back at work. We chatted for a long time and when she showed me what her reconstruction looked like, I couldn't believe it. I thought that I had the wrong person because it looked marvellous. I knew then that was the choice for me.

To those who are not sure whether to talk to other patients, I would say that it is a 'must'. I now speak to other patients myself. They tell me that they want to know how it actually is, how they are going to feel each day, how long before they will feel better, what to take into hospital and what they can or can't do afterwards. If I meet them, I show them my reconstructed breasts as well. When they get to the stage of nipples, they pop round again to have another look.

It does help to allay worries by talking to someone who has had the surgery before. I did want to have a look at someone else but wouldn't have wanted to have it forced on me. I was glad to know what to expect before the operation. That helped me to be comfortable with it. "

" I did not talk to anyone who had already had breast reconstruction, although I was told that there was a group that met near my home, where I could talk with someone who had gone through it. In hindsight, it probably would have helped me to have seen a finished reconstruction. You don't look any different. I was apprehensive about looking at the breast after the operation but after I had looked, I felt much better. Don't worry if you would prefer not to take up this option if it is offered. "

I didn't talk to anyone who had the operation beforehand as I didn't want to frighten myself with someone else's experience. At the end of the day, whatever happened to me was going to happen and how I dealt with it was down to me. 〃

Libraries and bookshops

Most libraries can get a comprehensive selection of books on breast disease if you ask them, at no cost to yourself.

Internet websites

You may be able to find some very useful information on the Internet, but do remember that it's often very detailed and may not reflect what your own surgeon is able to do for you. It's also possible to use the Internet to exchange thoughts and questions with other patients.

〃 I read as much information as I could get my hands on and the plastic surgeon told me about websites to look at. I was told to bear in mind that only the best results would be on there. I also discussed it with my family. I wondered how on earth I was going to make the decision. I was lucky enough to speak to two women who had the breast reconstructions I was considering. That was very helpful. 〃

17 Final comments – Would I do it again?

Making your mind up about breast reconstruction can be a long and difficult process. Not everyone will decide that breast reconstruction is for them. Taking time to look at all the possibilities and the practical implications will help to reassure you that you've made the right decision. Talking to your team, other patients and those close to you will help to clarify your thoughts and make your decision easier.

Here are some final thoughts from people who have been through this process and made their decisions, and who've had time to reflect on the results.

Differing views about the timing of breast reconstruction

“ I would urge women to go for immediate breast reconstruction if it is offered because to go back for a reconstruction after mastectomy would be daunting. If you are able to come out of surgery feeling feminine, able to wear nice swimsuits and go into a public changing room without worrying, this is great. Also, I wanted to be able to cuddle my grandchildren and didn't want to be a different shape for them. ”

“ I feel that I made the right decision about delaying the reconstruction. Things happened so quickly and I don't think that I could have made a decision about reconstruction as well at the time. I knew that the opportunity would still be there for me in the future. It was important to me that I wasn't shutting the door on it. ”

Immediate reconstruction was not an option because of other treatments

" The surgeon wouldn't do breast reconstruction at the same time as the mastectomy, mainly because they didn't know what sort of treatment I was going to need afterwards, particularly radiotherapy. That was fine for me. Personally, it would have been too much to have it all done at once.

Which reconstruction you have is a personal choice. The DIEP flap is a big operation and wouldn't be everyone's choice but it was the right one for me. I didn't realise the scrutiny that I would be under in the High Dependency Unit after the operation, which can be a bit frightening, but the care I had was excellent and each day was an improvement. I didn't talk to anyone who had the operation beforehand as I didn't want to frighten myself with someone else's experience. At the end of the day, whatever happened to me was going to happen and how I dealt with it was down to me. The operation was a huge success and has given me back my confidence. "

Appearance after breast reconstruction

" It is over two years since the operation and I feel fine about my appearance. It's not too great when I am stripped off but when you are 60, it's not too great anyway. I don't feel conscious of it at all when I am dressed and I don't think that anyone notices, even though my breasts are not quite level. My husband is quite happy about it because the bottom line is that I am still here and that is the important thing as far as he is concerned.

The big bonus about reconstruction is that if you do a lot of swimming, or when you go on holiday, you don't have to think about a swimming costume. I still wear the same style that I wore before the surgery. After reconstruction, you do want to wear bras that are nice. You have a cleavage and can take the neckline of clothes down a bit. You want to feel attractive again and it can be done. The fact that the breasts are different only matters between yourself and your partner. As long as the relationship is working, then it is not a problem.

I know that I have been lucky and it could have been so much worse to lose something else. We decided that the breast was really only there for the children and as a sex object. When you get older, it is less important and has done its function. If anyone chopped my right hand off, then my life would change. Losing my breast has not changed my life.
"

" The reconstruction itself looks brilliant and that is a combination of the surgeon's skill and the fact that I kept my own skin and nipple. I am really proud of it and don't think that I shall ever take my body for granted. I don't feel any less confident than I was before. If anything, I feel more confident about myself now. I was determined not to be beaten by any of it – the cancer as well as the operation. I did not want to be the victim and I think that was helpful.
"

" It is ten years since my reconstruction was done and I am glad that I had it done. I have seen ladies since then who have had a mastectomy and reconstruction at the same time and they were fantastic. I could not see which one had been reconstructed. It was different for me but I am happy. I hope that my husband still loves me, not for my breasts but for who I am. He has never told me that he doesn't like the reconstruction. At the same time, you just try to look after your appearance and do the best with what you have. As you get older, sex is still important but it is more about love, respect and caring.

People should not be scared of having breast reconstruction. It gives you a breast, femininity and confidence.
"

Positive comments about breast reconstruction, despite complications

" It took two years to fully recover from the reconstruction and the hernia repair. Nearly three years have passed since the reconstruction and I feel really good. I do feel that it has been worth having the reconstruction, despite the hernia.

When the hernia got bad, I wondered why I had bothered with the reconstruction but now I would say that it was definitely the right way to go. I would never have gone back for the reconstruction later if I had just had a mastectomy. Nobody would ever know that I have had a reconstruction and I haven't got an implant – that was something that I didn't want. It is just all me and really good. I don't have any problems with wearing swimming costumes and as I am too old to wear bikinis, the square tummy button doesn't matter either.

I know of others who have had complications after reconstruction and I don't think that any of them would have done things differently. It was well worth it.

Coping with having both breasts reconstructed

It may be easier to accept mastectomies and reconstructions when both sides are involved because I have nothing left to remind me of what I had. It was traumatic at the time but easier later. The reconstructions have given me so much confidence, which I didn't think I would get back after the mastectomies. Even if there are a few drawbacks at the time of surgery, reconstruction changes your attitude to everything.

Re-evaluating priorities

The whole experience has made me re-evaluate my priorities. I did appreciate things before and didn't take things for granted but now, even more so, I consider myself so lucky and appreciate things in sharp contrast. It has made me realise what is important.

You have to learn to be kind to yourself. Looking back on my working routine before the diagnosis, I wasn't being fair to myself. That is something that I am more aware of.

The reconstruction has given me a very natural appearance. I am confident in my dress and day-to-day life. If I had to, I would do the same again.

Would you recommend breast reconstruction to others?

" I would recommend reconstruction but it is a personal choice and it depends on how you can cope mentally with not having a breast. I would look and ask whether it is worth the pain of a long operation. It was worth it for me. You can go back to normal life afterwards. I look in the mirror and everything is fine. I feel like me and that is life as it should be. I have never looked back. There is light at the end of the tunnel. "

" I would say to someone considering reconstruction to do it. It makes you continue to feel like a woman and you also only have to go through it once. The whole experience has made me think that I should stop and live for today. Obviously we all hope that we won't have to face it but having done so, you have to be as positive as possible. There were days when I thought that it was horrible and didn't know how to go on but I talked myself through it and got on again. You should take the opportunities that you are given so that you can come out feeling as complete a woman as you can. "

Deciding reconstruction is not for you

" Having got myself so that I am comfortable after mastectomy, I don't particularly want the body change that a reconstruction would bring. I am also scared of playing about with what I have got. I have got one breast and that is fine. I would not want to end up looking at a reconstructed breast and thinking that actually I prefer what I had before. "

" It is a year since the operation (mastectomy) and I am happy and comfortable with it. It is part of how things are and that is it. I have achieved my aim of going back to work and getting on with life. I do have times when I feel down about it but would not want reconstruction now because I would rather avoid operations if possible. "

" I was 50 when I chose to have a mastectomy, rather than a lumpectomy and radiotherapy. I did not know anyone who had had breast cancer before, so had no pre-conceived ideas. My decision was made partly because I did not want to have radiotherapy but also because I thought that I didn't have the need for the breast any more. I just wanted to get rid of it and get on with life. Breast reconstruction was mentioned to me but I was quite happy not to have it. The loss of a breast did not concern me. I am a country person, not a fashion person, so not having a cleavage didn't worry me. My husband was very happy to go along with this decision.

I think that it is very important to be very open and talk about the mastectomy. I talked with my husband a lot. I did joke with very close friends and a sense of humour helps. It is good to take each day as it comes, be positive and do the exercises. It is important to get on with it because you have been given another chance. "

The very personal nature of decisions about reconstruction is reflected in the range and diversity of these thoughts. They highlight the importance of looking carefully at your own priorities and lifestyle before making up your mind about breast reconstruction. Taking time now to consider all your options is a very worthwhile investment for the future – so that you'll be happy with whatever choice you make.

Useful contacts and sources of information

Finding out about breast surgeons and clinics

The Association of Breast Surgery at BASO

Professional representative body for breast and oncoplastic surgeons in the UK (based at the Royal College of Surgeons of England). It provides a list of surgeons specialising in the management of breast conditions, including breast cancer.

The Association of Breast Surgery at BASO
The Royal College of Surgeons of England
35–43 Lincoln's Inn Fields
London WC2A 3PE
Tel: 020 7869 6852
Fax: 020 7404 6574
Email: lucydavies@baso.org.uk
Website: www.baso.org.uk

British Association of Plastic Reconstructive and Aesthetic Surgeons

Professional representative body for plastic and reconstructive surgeons in the UK (based at the Royal College of Surgeons of England). It provides advice on the management of conditions and information about the work of the surgeons and how to find a surgeon.

The British Association of Plastic Reconstructive and
Aesthetic Surgeons
The Royal College of Surgeons
35–43 Lincoln's Inn Fields
London WC2A 3PE
Tel: 020 7831 5161
Fax: 020 78314041
Email: secretariat@bapras.org.uk
Website: www.bapras.org.uk

Dr Foster

Independent information on health services in your area, including details of waiting lists and doctors who might be treating you.

Website: www.drfoster.co.uk/public.asp

National organisations providing advice and information

Breakthrough Breast Cancer

The UK's leading charity committed to fighting breast cancer through research, campaigning and education.

Freephone information line: 08080 100 200
Website: www.breakthrough.org.uk

Breast Cancer Care

The UK's leading charity for breast cancer support and detailed information. Services include a telephone helpline, a forum for younger women, an online chat forum and a prosthesis fitting service.

Breast Cancer Care
5–13 Great Suffolk Street
London SE1 0NS
Tel: 0845 092 0800
Helpline: 0808 800 6000 (textphone: 0808 800 6001)
Ask the Nurse Service: email info@breastcancercare.org.uk
Website: www.breastcancercare.org.uk

Breast Cancer Care (Scotland)

4th Floor
40 Enoch Square
Glasgow G1 4DH
Helpline: 0808 800 6000
Email: sco@breastcancercare.org.uk
Website: www.breastcancercare.org.uk

Cancerbackup

Europe's leading cancer information service with up-to-date cancer information, practical advice and support for cancer patients, their families and their carers.

Cancerbackup
3 Bath Place
Rivington Street
London EC2A 3JR
Tel: 020 7696 9003
Cancer information helpline: 0808 800 1234 (freephone),
020 7739 2280 (standard rate)
Website: www.cancerbackup.org.uk (including email link for queries)

Cancer Help UK

A free information service about cancer and cancer care provided by Cancer Research UK for people with cancer or their families.

Tel: 0808 800 4040 (freephone)
Website: www.cancerhelp.org.uk

DIPEX

Directory of Patient Experiences
Website: www.dipex.org

Macmillan Cancer Support

Provides practical, medical, emotional and financial support as well as listing support and self-help groups.

Macmillan Cancer Support
89 Albert Embankment
London SE1 7UQ
Head office (London) tel: 020 7840 7840
Fax: 020 7840 7841
Macmillan cancerline: 0808 808 2020
Email: cancerline@macmillan.org.uk
Website: www.macmillan.org.uk

Suppliers of bras, clothes, swimwear and prostheses

Amoena (UK) Ltd

Provides specialist mastectomy bras, swimwear and prostheses Mail order as well as fitting service and shop in Chandlers Ford, Hampshire (appointment needed).

Tel: 0800 072 8866 (freephone)
08000726636 (orders)
Email: agmaor@amoena.com
Website: www.amoena.co.uk

Anita UK Ltd

Specialist bras, swimwear and prostheses available in some shops. Range listed on website.

Tel: 0207435 2258
Email: anita.gb@anita.net
Website: www.anita.com

Bravissimo

Larger cup sizes in bras and swimwear, as well as some clothing. Catalogue, mail order, online shop and some high street shops.

Tel: 01926 459859
Website: www.bravissimo.com

Contura Belle (Thamert/Silima)

Specialist bras, swimwear, accessories and prostheses. Catalogue, mail order, online shop.

Tel: 01295 257 422
Email: info@conturabelle.co.uk
Website: www.conturabelle.co.uk

Eloise

Specialist and unpocketed bras, swimwear, clothes, prostheses, accessories. Catalogue, mail order, online shop, shop with fitting service (Bury St Edmonds, Suffolk).

Tel: 0845 225 5080
Email: sales@eloise.co.uk
Website: www.eloise.co.uk

Little Women

Small cup sized bras and swimwear. Catalogue, mail order, online shop.

Tel: 01455 274411
Email: enquiries@littlewomen.co.uk
Website: www.littlewomen.co.uk

Nicola Jane

High-quality post-mastectomy fashion offering bras, prostheses and swimwear. Items can be bought online, via a catalogue, or in person at one of their three shops, which have fitting services.

Tel: 0845 095 2121 (UK order line)
Tel: 020 7253 7841 (London shop)
Tel: 01243 533188 (Chichester shop)
Tel: 0113 258 7900 (Leeds shop at Oops and Downes)
Email: info@nicolajane.com
Website: www.nicolajane.com

Royce Lingerie Ltd

Pocketed and unpocketed (non-wired) bras. Catalogue, online shop only.

Tel: 01295 265557
Email: sales@royce-lingerie.co.uk
Website: www.royce-lingerie.co.uk

Trulife

Mastectomy bras, accessories and prostheses. Catalogue, mail order.

Tel:0800 716770 (freephone)
Website: www.trulife.co.uk/womenshealthcare.html

Womanzone

Specialist, made-to-measure swimwear, as well as bras, accessories and prostheses. Catalogue, mail order, online shop, shop with fitting service in Warrington, Cheshire.

Tel: 01925 768992
Email: sales@woman-zone.co.uk
Website: www.woman-zone.co.uk

Physiotherapy/exercises

Fighting Breast Cancer – We Can Help

Presented by Eleanor Meade with Rosemary Conley. Compassion Production Limited, 2003.

Exercise video/DVD designed especially for women who have had breast reconstruction. The exercises are performed by Rosemary Conley, and the video comes in sections covering relevant exercises following different types of reconstruction. There's an additional video in the pack that contains a series of testimonies from a variety of women who have undergone mastectomy and reconstruction. The women and their partners talk frankly and openly about all aspects of treatment, from telling their families, to coping with surgery and chemotherapy, to life afterwards.

Ordering information can be found at **www.compassion.co.uk** or email **sales@compassion.co.uk**. or phone **0845 226 9470**.

Glossary

Anaesthetist   A doctor who will give you medicine that will put you to sleep during an operation

Analgesic   Pain-relieving medicine

Apex   The most prominent part of the breast

Areola   The pigmented area of skin around the nipple

Arrow flap   A type of nipple reconstruction

Aspirate   To draw off with a syringe

Atheroma   Fatty deposits which clog arteries

Augmentation mammoplasty   Cosmetic procedure to increase your breast size using a breast implant

Autologous reconstruction   Building a new breast using only your own tissue without the need for an implant or a tissue expander

Auto-transfusion   Blood transfusion where your own blood has been stored and is transfused back to you

Axilla   Armpit

Bilateral mastectomy   An operation to remove both breasts

Bipedicled TRAM flap   Breast reconstruction using both of your rectus abdominus muscles and tissue in the abdomen

Body image   The internal view a person has of their body

Breast implant   A synthetic device (usually made partly of silicone) that is put into your breast to enlarge it or replace tissue which has been surgically removed

Breast reconstruction   An operation to rebuild your breast and restore what disease and surgery have taken away as realistically as possible

Breast reduction   An operation to reduce your breast size

Breast screening   Checking your breast, usually with mammograms or ultrasound scans to look for early breast problems

Capsular contracture   A scar or hard shell of tissue forming around a breast implant

Cellulitis   Spreading infection of the skin

Chemotherapy   Anti-cancer drugs

Chromosome   Part of a cell nucleus responsible for the transmission of hereditary characteristics

Clinical trials   Research studies used to compare two or more treatments to help find new or improved treatments

Comfy   A soft, light pad that is often worn after a mastectomy, while the scar is still healing, to restore body shape and give confidence before it is possible to wear a silicone prosthesis to replace the breast

Cosmetic augmentation   An operation to use breast implants to increase breast volume and enhance the bust

CV flap   A type of nipple reconstruction

DIEP flap (deep inferior epigastric artery perforator flap)   A type of breast reconstruction using tissue from your abdomen

Donor site   The space left behind once the muscle has been moved

Drainage tubes   Small tubes placed in an operation site that help to drain any fluid away and keep the area dry to promote healing

Ductal carcinoma in situ (DCIS)   A pre-cancerous change in breast cells

Delayed breast reconstruction   Surgically rebuilding a breast months or years after a mastectomy

DNA   Deoxyribonucleic acid (your genetic 'fingerprint')

Exchange of implant   An operation to remove a breast implant already in place and replace it with something similar that may give you a better shape

Fat necrosis   The death of fatty tissue due to trauma or lack of blood supply

Free flap/free tissue transfer/microvascular flap   Tissue that is moved to another site in the body having been disconnected from its original blood supply. It is then reconnected to a blood supply in its new location

Genetic code   The part of your gene which contains your genetic fingerprint

Glandular tissue   Breast tissue

Graft take   The ability of the skin graft to pick up its new blood supply and thrive

Haematoma   A collection of blood building up around your operation site

High Dependency Unit   A hospital ward where patients are looked after when they need intensive monitoring or nursing care

Hormone therapy   Using medicines known to block or stop the production of hormones which may be encouraging the cancer to grow

Human genetic fingerprint   The pattern of molecules in the DNA which makes up your genes which is unique to every human

Hypertrophic scars   Raised, thickened and red scars

IGAP flap (inferior gluteal artery perforator flap)   Breast reconstruction using free flaps of skin and fat from the buttocks

Immediate breast reconstruction   Rebuilding your breast at the same time as the mastectomy

Inframammary fold   The crease at the bottom of your breast where it joins the chest wall

Injection valve/port   Part of a tissue expander which is used to inject saline into the expander

Keloid scars   Scars which continue to thicken and do not settle down

Lactiferous ducts   Ducts which pass through the glandular breast tissue and the nipple. They transport milk as well as providing projection for the nipple

LTT flap (lateral transverse thigh flap)   Free flap breast reconstruction using the 'saddlebag' area of the thighs

Latissimus dorsi (LD) reconstruction   A way of rebuilding your breast using an implant or tissue expander combined with part of your latissimus dorsi muscle

Lipofilling   A type of fat transfer

Lower pole of the breast   The part of the breast below the nipple

Lumpectomy   Removal of a cancerous lump from your breast

Lymphoedema   Swelling of your tissues when fluid from the lymphatic system gets trapped and cannot escape

Magnetic resonance imaging (MRI)   Using the magnetic properties of your tissues to build up detailed pictures of your anatomy

Mammogram   An x-ray of your breast

Mastectomy   An operation to remove a breast

Mastopexy   An operation to lift the breast

Maturation   The healing process of a scar over several months until it is blended into the surrounding tissue

Montgomery's tubercles   Glands that secrete a waxy fluid to moisturise and protect the nipple and areola

Mutation   A change or alteration of your genes

Myocutaneous muscle flap   Tissue made up of muscle, fatty tissue and skin that can be moved from one part of your body to another to reconstruct a breast

Neuro-vascular pedicle   The blood vessels and nerves which keep the flap alive

Nipple-areola complex (NAC)   Both your nipple and the surrounding area of pigmented skin (areola)

Nipple reconstruction   Rebuilding your nipple surgically

Oncologist   A doctor specialising in medical treatments for cancer

Oncoplastic surgeon   A surgeon trained in both cancer surgery and breast reconstruction

Partial mastectomy   An operation to remove a large amount of breast tissue

Pathologist   A doctor trained to analyse diseased tissue and body samples.

Patient-controlled analgesia   A machine used to give pain-killing medicines after an operation that a patient can control themselves

Pectoralis major muscle   A large triangular muscle lying over the front of your rib cage

Pedicled TRAM flap   Moving lower abdominal tissue into the breast area still attached to its original blood supply

Perforators   Small branches of blood vessels

Physiotherapy   Exercises and advice given to help regain normal movement in all areas affected by an operation, medical treatment or disease

Prosthesis   A synthetic breast-form designed to fit into a bra to replace either your whole breast or part of it

Ptosis   Natural drooping of the breast

Radiotherapy   High-energy x-ray treatment used to damage cancer cells and stop them dividing

Rectus abdominus muscle   A muscle in your abdominal wall

Reduction mammoplasty   A breast reduction combined with a breast lift

Risk-reducing mastectomy   An operation to remove a healthy breast when it proven that there is a high risk of disease occurring in the future

Rough surface texturing   A process to make the surface of a breast implant rough rather than smooth to cut down the scar tissue reaction around the implant

Rubens flap   Breast reconstruction using a free flap from the fat deposits over your hips, the 'love handles'

Saline   A sterile salt solution, with the same salt content as body fluids

Septicaemia   Blood poisoning

Seroma   A collection of fluid that accumulates in the spaces left behind after surgery

SGAP (superior gluteal artery perforator flap)   Breast reconstruction using free flaps of skin and fat from your buttocks

Silicones   Synthetic materials built around a frame of silicon and oxygen atoms

Silicone elastomer   Silicone rubber

Silicone gel bleeding   The leakage of silicone gel through an intact outer shell

Skate flap   A type of nipple reconstruction

Skin and tissue expansion   Gradually stretching the skin and surrounding tissues with an adjustable implant to enlarge the area

Skin flap   A flap of tissue made up of skin, fat and blood vessels that can be moved to a nearby part of the body

Skin island   The skin that is attached to a flap when it is moved from the back or stomach to reconstruct the breast

Skin necrosis   Loss of healthy skin and fatty tissue due to a poor blood supply

Skin-sparing mastectomy   An operation to remove only breast tissue, preserving the whole skin envelope to provide cover for the new breast

Softie   A soft first prosthesis worn after mastectomy – see 'comfy'

Sub-cuticular sutures   Stitches placed just underneath the outer layer of your skin that don't need to be removed

Subglandular   Under the breast tissue

Submuscular   Under a muscle

Subpectoral   Under the pectoralis muscle

Superficial epigastric vessels   Blood vessels supplying the wall of the lower abdomen

Superior epigastric vessels   Blood vessels coming out of the chest and nourishing the muscles in your abdominal wall

Suture   Stitch

Tattoo   The use of pigments to colour the skin and enhance the nipple reconstruction

Temporary expander   An implant used to stretch the tissues that can be replaced with a breast implant if necessary

Thrombosis   Blood clot

Tissue expander   An expandable bag that can be placed under the skin and gradually increased in size to make the surrounding tissues stretch

TRAM flap (transverse rectus abdominus myocutaneous flap)   Method of breast reconstruction using tissue and muscle from the abdomen

TUG flap (transverse upper gracilis flap)   Breast reconstruction using free muscle flaps from the inner aspects of your thighs

Unipedicled TRAM flap   Breast reconstruction using one of your two rectus abdominus muscles and tissue from your abdominal wall

Urinary catheter   A small tube placed into your bladder to drain urine

Volume displacement   Replacing tissue that has been removed with tissue borrowed from another part of the same breast

Volume replacement   Replacing tissue that has been removed with tissue borrowed from another part of your body

Index

Numbers *in italics* denote illustrations.

abdominal hernias 19, 83, *83*, 84, 88
abdominal tissue, use of 2, 15, 19
  see DIEP flaps; TRAM flaps
abscesses 139
age 14, 15, 109
areola, the 115, *116*
  skin grafting 119, 122, *122*, 126
  tattooing *10*, 37, 120, 122–3, *123*, *124*, 125, 126
armpit (axilla) 53, 62, 67, 87
  see also lymph glands
arms 91, 92, 94, 173, 174, 175, 177–8
  loss of movement 113, 176, 179
  lymphoedema *144*, 144–5
  numbness 93, 112
  postoperative exercising 93, 95, 112, 170–71, *172*, 173, 178, 199
arrow flaps 121, *121*
asymmetry
  natural 136
  see symmetry surgery
atheroma 139
augmentation *see* breast enlargement
autologous LD flap
  reconstruction 16, 19, 51, 61–3, *62*, *64*
  advantages and disadvantages 68–9, 72
  comparison with implant-based reconstruction 45, 55, 58–9, 72
  delayed 61, 63, *63*, 66

effect on back muscles 66–7, 69, 70
  length of operation 66
  and need for physiotherapy 66
  and 'patch effects' 12, 68, *69*
  patients' experiences 62, 66–7, 69–71, 167
  recovery period 66–7, 175–6
  success rate 67
  see also symmetry surgery
autotransfusions 80

back muscles, use of *see* autologous *and* implant-based LD flap reconstruction; volume replacement procedures
Becker tissue expander 20, *33*
bilateral risk reducing
  mastectomies *10*, 20, 49, 61, 128–30, *129*, *140*, 153, *153*, 155–6
  patients' experiences 156–60, 212
biopsies
  sentinel node 52, 145
  waiting for results 108, 109
blood clots 88, 138, *see also* haematomas
blood-thinning injections 80, 138
blood transfusions 80, 141
bras 41, 65, 92, 113, 134, 163–4
  mastectomy 47, 193, 194, 195–7
breast care nurses/team 6, 8, 16, 60, 111, 162, 190, 194, 206

breast enlargement
(augmentation) 24, 27–8, 37,
128, *135*, 135–6, *136*
breast lifts (mastopexies) 37, 57,
61, 64, 128, 130, 130–31
breast reconstruction 2–3
and coping with emotions
185–6
number of operations
needed 14–15, 165
options 15–16, *see*
decision-making
preparing for 173–4
and realistic expectations
185
see also delayed *and*
immediate breast
reconstruction
breast reduction
and partial mastectomies
106–7
patients' experiences 132–4
for symmetry 20–21, 37, 57,
58, *65*, 128, *131*, 131–2
breasts, other (normal)
matching 37, 192–3, *see*
breast enlargement;
breast lifts; breast
reduction; symmetry
surgery and reducing risk
of cancer *see* bilateral
mastectomies
bruising 11, 140, *141*, 165
buttocks, using tissue from 15, *see*
SGAP flaps

cancer
effects of reconstruction on
14
genes and genetic testing
for 151–5
see also bilateral risk-
reducing mastectomies
capsular contracture/capsules 36,
65, 42, 135
cartilage grafts (for nipples) 118,
122

catheters, urinary 13, 80
cellulitis 139
checkups 38
chemotherapy 5, 8, 47, 50, 82,
147, 149
children, reactions of 47, 158,
166–7, 188
'chromosome 17' 151
clothing 3, 5, 40, 42, 133, 183, 201
in hospital 163–4
see also bras; swimsuits
coldness, feeling of (in new breast)
3, 189
complications after surgery
58–9, 108, *83*, 83–4, 88,
125–6, 167
convalescence *see* recovery times
cosmetic breast implants 24,
27–8
CV flaps 120, *120*

decision-making 5–6, 8, 9,
13–14, 182–4, 203–4
and getting information 6,
204–6, 208, *see also* breast
care nurses
and other people 187–8
weighing up advantages and
disadvantages 6–8, 17–19,
72, 184
see also talking to other
patients
deep inferior epigastric vessels *74*,
86
see also DIEP flaps
dehydration 138
delayed breast reconstruction 4, 6,
8, 9, 14, 88, 184–5, 209, 210
autologous LD flap
reconstruction 63, *63*
and implants 28, 29
and scars 12
diabetics 75, 88
DIEP (deep inferior epigastric
artery perforator)
flaps 15, 19, 85, *86*, 86–8, *87*,
210

abdominal scar 85, *86*, *87*, *89*, 91, 92, 93
comparison with pedicled TRAM flaps 85–6, 96
complications 88, *see also* fat necrosis
patients' experiences 90–95
and radiotherapy *89*, 89–90
recovery time 12–13, 85, 87, 91, 92, 94–5, 171, 177–8
success rates 88, 97
and symmetry surgery 89
'donor sites' 12, 45
abdomen 45, 75, *75*, 77, 77–8, 88
back 16, 45, 66–7, 68–9, 70
buttocks 15, 96–7, *98*, 98
thighs 16, 97, *97*
drains/drainage *see* fluid drainage
driving 67, 81, 91, 95, 163, 166, 167, 171
droopy breasts, matching 37, 38, *50*, 90, 91, 130
ductal carcinoma in situ (DSIS) 8

emotions, coping with 157, 185–6, 206
enlarging breasts *see* breast enlargement
epigastric vessels *74*, *85*
exercise video/DVD 179
exercise(s) 165, 169–71, 172, 173
after implant surgery 35, 174–5
after LD flap surgery 66–7, 176
after mastectomies 199
after partial reconstruction 112, 113
after TRAM/DIEP surgery 177, 178
preoperative 173–4
expanders *see* tissue expanders

family history of cancer 20, 128–9, 154–5

see also genetic testing
fat necrosis 83, 88, 95, 149
fatty tissue, lipofilling with 64
FDA *see* Food and Drug Administration
femininity, loss of 13, 56, 181, 211, 213
'flap' operations 12–13, 15–16
see DIEP flaps; TRAM flaps
fluid drainage 13, 34–5, 36, 55, 56, 61, 67, 140, 162, 199
after mastectomies 198–9
follow-up visits 38
Food and Drug Administration (FDA) 26, 27
free tissue transfers 45, 68, 86–7

genes, cancer (BRCA1 and BRCA2) 151, 152, 153
genetic testing 151–5
golf, playing 53, 137, 176

haematomas 36, 59, 83, 88, 140–41
heart problems 51, 88
Herceptin 150
hernias 19, 83, *83*, 84, 88, 211–12
hormonal treatments 5, 149
hospital stays 163
clothing in 163–4
housework 171, 176
husbands and partners 111, 156, 158, 160, 187–8
see also sexual relationships
hydrotherapy 157

IGAP (inferior gluteal artery perforator) flaps 96
immediate breast reconstruction 3–4, 6, 28
advantages and disadvantages 7–9, 209
and effect on cancer 14
implant-based LD flap reconstruction 15, 45–6, 48, 49, *50*, 52, 53, 55–7, *57*

advantages and
  disadvantages 18, 60, 72
comparisons with
  autologous LD 45, 55,
  58, 72
complications 58–9
contraindicated 51–2
drainage of back wounds
  55, 56, 59, 61, 67–8, 70
exercises after 35, 174–5
and infection 59, 139
injection ports 53, 57, 133
inserting expander 56–7, 57
'marking up' for 53, 54
numbness and stiffness of
  back 66–7, 69, 70
patients' experiences 46,
  47–8, 49, 50–51, 56, 59–
  60, 166
recovery time 174–5
scarring of back 18, 55, 69
see also implants; tissue
  expanders
implants, subpectoral 15, 17, 23,
  24–5, 28, 29, 29–30
advantages and
  disadvantages 35–7
for breast enlargement 135,
  135–6
durability 37
patients' experiences 38–43
recovery period 30, 34–5,
  38–9
rupture of 37, 135–6
saline-filled 25, 26, 30, 53,
  57, 135
silicone 25–7
and silicone bleeding 36
see also implant-based LD
  reconstruction; tissue
  expanders
Independent Review Group (IRG)
  26
infections 35, 59, 88, 93, 138, 139,
  139, 141, 159
information, getting 161, 183,
  204–6

see also breast care nurses;
  talking to other patients
injection ports/valves 30, 31, 32,
  34, 53, 57, 133
Internet websites 208
IRG *see* Independent Review Group

lactiferous ducts 115, *116*
latissimus dorsi muscles *52*, 53, *62*,
  62–3
latissimus dorsi reconstruction 45,
  137
    see autologous LD
      reconstruction; implant-
      based LD reconstruction;
      volume replacement
      procedures
leg blood clots 138
lipofilling 64
liposuction 83
lopsidedness (of breasts) 36
    see symmetry surgery
LTT (lateral transverse thigh) flap 97
lumpectomies *see* partial
  mastectomies
lung problems 51, 88, 138
lymph glands 53, 143, 144
  and sentinel node biopsy 145
lymph nodes, examination of 36
lymphoedema 143–4
  of the arm *144*, 144–5
  of the breast 144

mammograms 20, 131, 136, 153
'marking up' 53, *54, 63, 64*
mastectomies 1, *192*, 194, *200*
  and clothing 193, *200*, 201,
    see also bras, mastectomy
  exercises after 199
  fluid drainage 198–9
  patients' experiences 191–2,
    194, 201–2
  psychological aspects 13,
    56, 181, 198
  recovery time 200–1
  risk-reducing *see* bilateral
    mastectomies

without reconstruction
191–2, 213–14
see also partial mastectomies;
prostheses
mastopexies *see* breast lifts
microvascular flaps 45
'miniflaps', LD myocutaneous
104, 105, *105*, *106*
monoclonal antibodies 150
Montgomery's tubercles 115, *116*
MRI (magnetic resonance
imaging) 153
myocutaneous flaps 44–5
see also 'miniflaps'

NAC (nipple–areola complex)
reconstruction 37, 115–16, *116*,
117–18, *124*
complications 125–6
patients' experiences 116–
17, 125, 126–7
see also areola; nipple
reconstruction; nipples
necrosis (skin death) 58–9
see also fat necrosis
nipple reconstruction *10*, 15, *47*,
118, *124*
arrow flap 121, *121*
cartilage grafts 118, 122
CV flap 120, *120*
skate flap 119, *119*
nipples 115, *116*
and breast reduction 132
prosthetic (false) 127, *127*
see also nipple
reconstruction
numbness
of backs 69, 70
of reconstructed breasts 3,
5, 11–12, 46, 143
nurses *see* breast care nurses

obesity/overweight 51, 67, 75,
138, 149
oncoplastic surgeons 103, 205, 206
outpatient visits 163
ovarian cancer 152

overexpansion of implants 32, *32*,
33

pain 34, 46, 49, 111, 162–3
pain relief 111, 138, 142–3, *143*,
163
partial mastectomies
(lumpectomies) 6, 49, 50, 102
after surgery 111–12
and breast reconstruction
103, 109, 110, *110*,
see volume displacement
and volume replacement
procedures
patients' experiences 109,
110–14
recovery time 111–14
partners *see* husbands and partners
'patch effects' 12, 68, *69*
patient-controlled analgesia (PCA)
80, 111, 142–3, *143*
PDMS (polydimethylsiloxane) 25
'peau d'orange' 144
pectoralis major muscle 15, 23, *24*
pedicles 44–5, 63, 78
pelvic tilting exercises 177
photographic records, keeping 187
physiotherapists/physiotherapy
13, 66, 84, 93, 165, 169–70, 174
pilates 172, *173*, 178
pneumonia 138
posture 170, 174–5, 178
prostheses, external 3, 14, 38, 47,
70, 102, 181, 193, 194, 195,
195, *200*
nipples 127, *127*
psychological effects 156, 180,
181–2, 185–6
see also femininity, loss of
psychological support 190
ptosis (droop) 38, *50*, 74, 130
questions, asking 3, 16, 49,
162–4
radiotherapy 5, 16, 49, 146, *147*,
149
effects on breast implants
48–9, 60, 65, 148

effects on reconstructed
breasts 14, 51, 60, 68,
89–90, 148, *148*, 149, 150
and lymphoedema 145
and NAC reconstruction
125, 126
and sentinel node biopsy 52
and timing of breast
reconstruction 8, 110, 147–8
records, keeping 186–7
recovery times 12–13, 34, 35, 157,
163, 167–8, 171
after mastectomies 200–1
*see also under specific
techniques*
rectus muscles 78, 79, 85, 86
Regional Specialist Genetics
Service 152
risk-reducing mastectomies *see*
bilateral mastectomies
rowing 18, 53, 95
'Rubens' flaps 97
running 35, 172, 173

saline-filled implants 25, 26, 30,
53, 57, 135
scars 3, 12, 19, 70–71, 139, *140*,
162
abdominal 19, 75, *75*, 77,
77–8, *87*, *89*, 177
on backs 18, 19, 53, *55*, 69
on breasts 17, 59
hypertrophic 139–40, *140*
and implants 35, 36
invisible 2, *2*, 10, *10*
keloid 140
massaging cream into 165,
177, 186
sensations in new breast 3, 5, 11–
12, 143, 162
sentinel node biopsies 52, 145
seromas 67–8, 70, 141–2, *142*
sexual relationships 94, 134, 156,
157, 181, 188–9, 210
SGAP (superior gluteal artery
perforator) flaps 96–7, *98*, 98,
99, 178–9

patients' experiences
99–101
shape of new breast 11, 53, 165
see also symmetry surgery
silicone implants 23, 25–7,
135–6
bleeding 36
leaking 37
temporary expanders 30
size of new breast 11, 20–21, 53,
60
see also symmetry surgery
skate flaps 119, *119*
skin death 58–9
skin 'expansion' 29–30
'skin islands' 12, *52*, 62, 63, 68, *69*,
104, *104*
sleeping difficulties 46, 51
smokers 58–9, 67, 75–6, 125, 138,
139, 149
sports 16, 18, 70, 172, 176, 183
stitches 34, 140, 162
stockings, compression 80, 138
subpectoral reconstruction *see*
implants; tissue expanders
support groups 206
surgeons 16, 19, 21–2, 97, 183,
205, 206
sutures *see* stitches
swelling after operation 11, 165
see also lymphoedema
swimming 47, 53, 134, 157, 172,
173, 176, 210
swimwear 3, 66, 196, 197
symmetry surgery 20–21, 57–8,
58, 64–5, *65*, 89–90

talking to other patients 16, 56,
109, 156, 185, 194, 206–8
tamoxifen 153
tattooing, areola *10*, 15, 37, 118,
120, 122–3, *123*, *124*, 125, 126
topup 123, *124*
tennis 172
thighs, using tissue from 16, 97–8,
97
thrombosis 138

timing of breast reconstruction
3–4, 6
see delayed *and* immediate
breast reconstruction
tiredness, post-operative 81, 158,
165, 166, 171
tissue expanders 11, 23, *29*, 29–30,
45
Becker 20, *33*, 41–2
inserting under LD flap
56–7, *57*
and overexpansion 32, *32*, *33*
permanent 30–32, *31*, *32*
rupture of 59
temporary 30, 32
see also implant-based LD
reconstruction; implants
TRAM (transverse rectus
abdominus myocutaneous) flaps
73
free *see* DIEP, IGAP *and* SGAP
flaps; pedicled *see below*
TRAM flap reconstruction,
pedicled 15, 19, 45, 51, 73–6,
74, *79*
and abdominal scar 75, *75*,
77, 77–8
comparison with DIEP flap
85–6, 96

complications *83*, 83–4
delayed 77, *78*, 78–9
failure rates 83
immediate 75, 77–8
length of operation 74, 80
patients' experiences 76–7,
80–82, 84, 167
recovery time 12–13, 78,
79–82, 84, 167, 177–8
unipedicled 79
TUG (transverse upper gracilis)
flap 97–8, *97*

valves, injection *see* injection
ports/valves
volume displacement procedures
104, 106–7
complications 108
numbness after 113
volume replacement procedures
104–6
complications 108
sensations after 112–13

work, returning to 92, 133, 157,
163, 172, 200–1

yoga 172, 173

Have you found **Breast Reconstruction – Your Choice** useful and practical? If so, you may be interested in other books from **Class Publishing**.

Breast Cancer: Answers at your fingertips

Val Speechley, Emma Pennery and Maxine Rosenfield

£14.99

Breast cancer affects the lives of millions of women, and strikes at the very heart of their self-image and identity. Not many people realise it can also affect men.

With earlier diagnosis and advances in treatment, many people live with breast cancer, or with the possibility of recurrence, for many years. This book, with its appealing question and answer format, provides sensitive information on all aspects of living with breast cancer.

Type 1 Diabetes: Answers at your fingertips
Type 2 Diabetes: Answers at your fingertips

Dr Charles Fox and Dr Anne Kilvert

£14.99

The latest edition of our bestselling reference guide on diabetes has now been split into two books covering the two distinct forms of the disease. These books maintain the popular question and answer format to provide practical advice for patients on every aspect of living with the condition.

'I have no hesitation in commending this book.' – Sir Steve Redgrave, Vice President, Diabetes UK

Dump Your Toxic Waist!

Dr Derrick Cutting

£14.99

The easy, drug-free and medically accurate way to lose inches, beat diabetes and stop that heart attack.

'… an excellent book for those who are interested in unclogging their arteries, or getting down to their ideal weight for good, or controlling their blood pressure, or discovering a new vitality' – The Family Heart Digest

Migraine – Answers at your fingertips

Dr Manuela Fontebasso

£14.99

Written by an experienced GP with a special interest in headache and migraine, this book acknowledges the uniqueness of every sufferer's experience. Communication between patient and professional is crucial if this complex condition is to be addressed and the best treatment prescribed.

This book will help you understand the nature of your headache, and give you the confidence to be involved in all areas of decision making.

Menopause – Answers at your fingertips

Dr Heather Currie

£17.99

The average age of the menopause is 51 years, but it can occur much earlier or later. The symptoms vary widely in their severity, and can include hot flushes, night sweats, palpitations, insomnia, joint pain and headaches. Women are at greater risk of osteoporosis after the menopause.

This invaluable guide answers hundreds of questions from women approaching or experiencing the menopause, and provides positive, practical advice on a range of issues.

Beating Depression

Dr Stefan Cembrowicz and Dr Dorcas Kingham

£17.99

Depression is one of most common illnesses in the world – affecting up to one in four people at some time in their lives. This book shows sufferers and their families that they are not alone, and offers tried and tested techniques for overcoming depression.

'All you need to know about depression, presented in a clear, concise and readable way.' – Ann Dawson, World Health Organization

PRIORITY ORDER FORM

Cut out or photocopy this form and send it (post free in the UK) to:

**Class Publishing Priority Service, FREEPOST 16705,
Macmillan Distribution, Basingstoke, RG21 6ZZ
Tel: 01256 302 699   Fax: 01256 812 558**

**Please send me urgently (tick below)
Post included price per copy (UK only)**

☐ **Breast Reconstruction – Your Choice** (ISBN 978 1 85959 197 0)   **£22.99**

☐ **Breast Cancer: Answers at your fingertips** (ISBN 978 1 85959 198 7)   **£17.99**

☐ **Type 1 Diabetes: Answers at your fingertips** (ISBN 978 1 85959 175 8)   **£17.99**

☐ **Type 2 Diabetes: Answers at your fingertips** (ISBN 978 1 85959 176 5) **£17.99**

☐ **Migraine: Answers at your fingertips** (ISBN 978 1 85959 170 3)   **£17.99**

☐ **Menopause: Answers at your fingertips** (ISBN 978 1 85959 155 0)   **£20.99**

☐ **Dump Your Toxic Waist!** (ISBN 978 1 85959 191 8)   **£17.99**

☐ **Beating Depression** (ISBN 978 1 85959 150 5)   **£20.99**

TOTAL: _____

Easy ways to pay:

Cheque: I enclose a cheque payable to Class Publishing for:

Credit card: please debit my ☐ Mastercard ☐ Visa ☐ Amex

Number: _____ Expiry date: _____

Name: _____

My address for delivery is: _____

_____

Town _____

County _____ Postcode _____

Telephone number (in case of query) _____

Credit card billing address if different from above _____

_____

Town _____

County _____ Postcode _____

Class Publishing's guarantee: remember that if, for any reason, you are not satisfied with these books, we will refund all your money, without any questions asked. Prices and VAT rates may be altered for reasons beyond our control.